I
Don't
Want
To
Settle

I Don't Want To Settle

Words for a lost generation

Dan Whitlam

Illustrated by Natti Shiner

First published in the UK in 2025 by Blink Publishing
An imprint of Bonnier Books UK
5th Floor, HYLO, 105 Bunhill Row,
London, EC1Y 8LZ

Copyright © Dan Whitlam, 2025
Illustrations Copyright © Natti Shiner, 2025

All rights reserved.

No part of this publication may be reproduced, stored or transmitted in
any form or by any means, electronic, mechanical, photocopying or otherwise,
without the prior written permission of the publisher.

The right of Dan Whitlam to be identified as Author of this work has been asserted by him in
accordance with the Copyright, Designs and Patents Act, 1988.

A CIP catalogue record for this book is available from the British Library.

Paperback ISBN: 9781785126260

Also available as an ebook and an audiobook

1 3 5 7 9 10 8 6 4 2

Design and Typeset by Envy Design Ltd
Printed and bound in Great Britain by Clays Ltd, Elcograf S.p.A.

Every reasonable effort has been made to trace copyright holders of
material reproduced in this book, but if any have been inadvertently
overlooked the publishers would be glad to hear from them.

This book is a work of Non-Fiction. Some names have been changed to
respect the privacy of those mentioned.

The authorised representative in the EEA is
Bonnier Books UK (Ireland) Limited.
Registered office address: Floor 3, Block 3, Miesian Plaza,
Dublin 2, D02 Y754, Ireland
compliance@bonnierbooks.ie

www.bonnierbooks.co.uk

For Hannah Whitlam.
I am because you were.

Contents

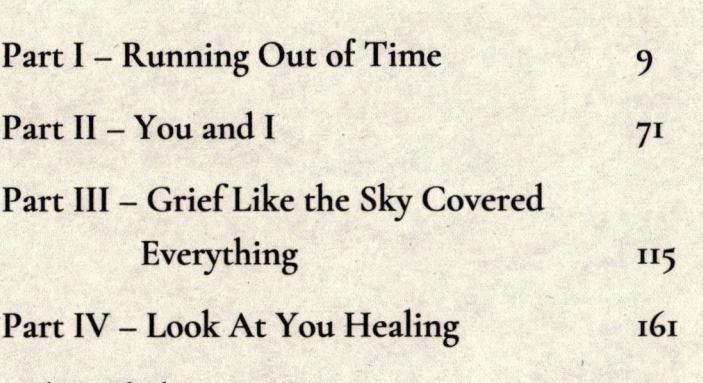

Part I – Running Out of Time   9

Part II – You and I   71

Part III – Grief Like the Sky Covered
           Everything   115

Part IV – Look At You Healing   161

Acknowledgements   207

Part I – Running Out of Time

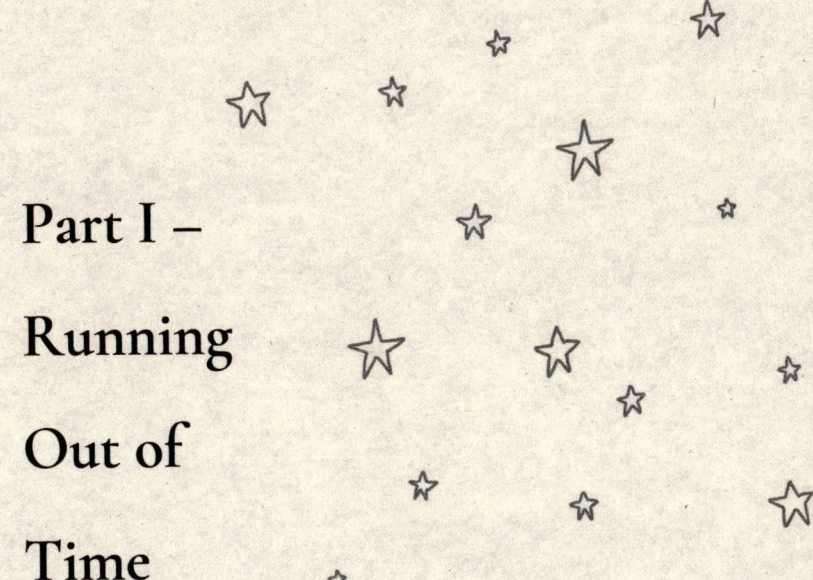

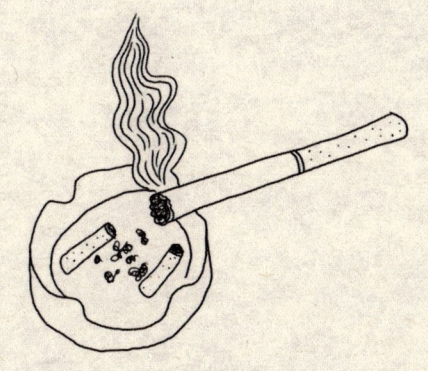

I Don't Want To Settle

My twenties have brought about a huge amount of anxiety surrounding choice.

What should I do with my life? How best to live it? Where can I achieve a satisfying balance of happiness and purpose?

For a lot of people, twenty-something is when you're given your first real taste of freedom – a chance to reinvent yourself and discover who you want to be, all while being bombarded with those dreaded questions:

'What do you want to do?'
'Are you happy?'
'Do you have a boyfriend/girlfriend?'
'Have you been promoted yet?'

A world of comparison and expectation leaves our twenties feeling less like an era of discovery and growth and more a case of: 'I'm running out of time.'

As I desperately tried to answer these questions and figure out my whole life and retirement plan before the age of 22-and-a-half, I was left overwhelmed, in a daze of overthinking.

What should I do? I wondered. *What am I good at?*

Everywhere we look, we are inundated with options and opinions. Videos circulate on social media of 19-year-olds who are supposedly multi-millionaires, telling you to buy into their get-rich-quick pyramid schemes and convincing us that selling dog beds on Amazon as a third-party seller could find you shacked up in Dubai, driving a white Ferrari.

I would, and often do, scroll for hours comparing my life to those presented to me via my phone, asking myself why I'm not as far along as they seem to be, ignoring how far I've come and how much I've achieved.

Comparison is the thief of joy, and I've certainly fallen to that trap many times. As I'm tucked up in bed, I tell myself that I'll be happier when I'm on a beach like that. Or when I have a job like them.

We're told we can do or be whatever we want. But this well-intentioned, supposedly freeing idea often leaves us feeling more overwhelmed than at ease. Consumed by the fear of making the wrong decision and the potential long-lasting consequences, we can be left in a state of paralysis that, at the time, feels safer than having to decide anything at all.

Too much to choose from, so I'll sit in my bed watching Friends *until I can try again tomorrow.*

It's dizzying: attempting to work out who you are but still making enough of a mark on the world to say, 'Look, Mum and Dad, I did a thing.' It took me a little while to get here, but I'd like to think my thing is writing.

I Don't Want To Settle

Putting my thoughts down into poems or short stories is what has helped me most when feeling lost. Writing from a place of lived truth or writing fictional/imagined scenarios has been a real escape for me. Of course, I understand we all have different lived experiences in our early adult life. Privilege and environment certainly play into all of this, but maybe a consistent takeaway is that perhaps we're all a bit lost? We're all figuring it out one day at a time and so, maybe, we can take solace in the fact we're doing it together? Maybe we're all exactly where we're meant to be? Maybe there's no right way of navigating life and so you should just do whatever feels right for you? I find I can explain myself better in moments of extremes through rhyme and romantic language, and I feel more in touch with myself when writing out what I'm going through, or what I've overcome. Maybe you can relate? I wrote this collection not just for myself as I went through times of pain and happiness, but also for anyone else who is feeling lost. I do hope you find reason, voice and a little comfort within these pages.

My poetry is by no means anywhere close to perfect, but I do think poetry and writing have the power to give reason to the reasonless and voice to the voiceless. And so this collection has not been written out of a deep need to share my writing purely with poetry lovers. Instead, I wanted to explore what it means to be young today, to truly grow into your adult self and feel like you're getting it wrong every single day. To identify what it's like to be moving through adulthood, where you may meet the love of your life at 10am, experience a devastating breakup at 1pm, then feel caught in a mental breakdown at 5pm, all in time to find peace and self-love again before bed at 10pm.

There are four parts to this book, four themes that I think best encapsulate what navigating life as a young adult has been like for me, and maybe for you, too. These were the shared experiences that kept coming up again and again for me as I wrote – the feelings and challenges my friends would talk about and seek counsel on, and which I would naturally gravitate to.

First up, a chapter on **Running Out of Time** – the panic years, the *Why do I feel everyone is ahead of me and I'm at a standstill?* dread. Then there's **You and I**, a chapter on love – both the romantic kind and the kind we show ourselves. **Grief Like the Sky Covered Everything** is about loss – the whirlwind of losing a partner, parent or friend. And then we come to **Look At You Healing**, a chapter on starting anew and being able to make peace with where you're at and what you've overcome.

If any of this rings true to you, then I hope you find some value in my words, even if it's only the realisation that, despite how it may feel at times, *you are not alone.*

I Don't Want To Settle

It's a false thought to young minds,
irony of being in your twenties but,
feeling like you're
running out of time.

A line we've all heard in this life of downers and daffodils,
find our highs in
ground
        down
                pills
and
cigarettes by the windowsill.

Still trying to fill your future with what
you should do.
Could do.
What your mum and dad would like you to.

When your mum and dad were sad as you
packed your bags cos
they frightened you.

You stub out your cigarette and take another sip of tequila
to kill the feeling that you should only go and think
in the future.

But
it's a rumour.
Nothing truer.
Wish I realised it sooner.

It's always sunny above the clouds.

So
live right here
for what's in front of you.

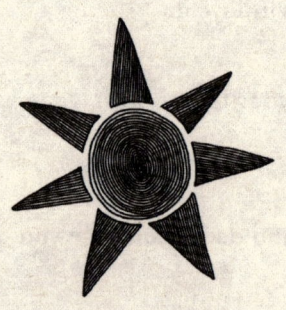

I Don't Want To Settle

You went to bed
with the dreams of
who you'd be in five years' time.

Not knowing that when you awoke
you were living the dreams
you'd had five years before.

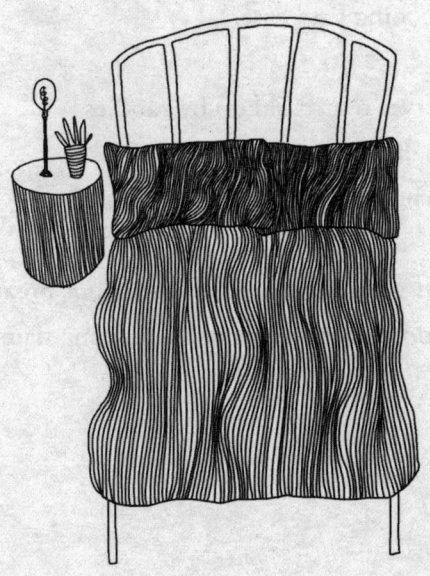

Dan Whitlam

 Enjoy the butterflies
for one day they'll give you their wings
and

leave.

Nerves will no longer be excitement without breath
just
an old friend you forget
that once lived inside of your chest.

First met on first dates
or
touching first base.

Nerves that build up by candles
when blowing out birthday cakes.
That learning phase.

Felt you turned a page when your breath broke quick
and hands held hot like a burning flame.

I Don't Want To Settle

Cos
you realised that nerves
just meant that you cared about something.
And they're not to be feared, but savoured.

So
notice those moments when you feel the
nerves settling in and sit with them.

Because once the nerves leave
it's hard to get that excitement back again.

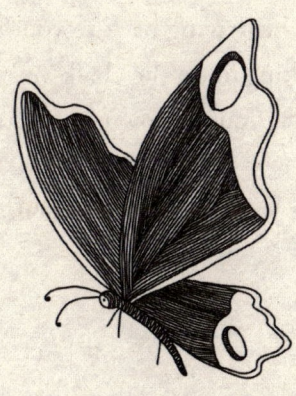

Dan Whitlam

Your dad used to mark your height
upon the side of the door.
Name scribbled in darker ink
next to lines of chalk.

He'd say, 'You're growing by the day, darling,
high above the floor.
And one day you'll witness the markings
of times that you were before.'

Now you've grown up, and grown on.

Moved that family house,
started your own one.
Living happily south of town.
But on days that you doubt yourself
you'll be driving back to your dad's.
Checking upon the chalk and
how far you've grown since little hands.

Oh, it was simpler back then.

Little

lines

I Don't Want To Settle

of

a

pen.

I should have sworn that I'd go to pause it,
to re-live again.
Certain feelings we cut on grass
while sitting with friends.
The ones who said it
that growing older is the start of the end.

Staring at when you were just a kid:
a line on the door.
Name scribbled in darker ink next to lines of chalk.
Dad said, 'You're growing by the day, darling,
high above the floor.'

So, look at what you've become.
You're this
and so much more.

Dan Whitlam

We were kids around a table just discussing a dream.
All asking *What do you wanna do?*
and *Who you pushing to be?*

Dad, he lifted his liquor, Mum was falling asleep.
We stayed awake with just the feeling
of following little dreams.

We'd try to catch it.
Open up our hands just to snatch it.
Hands would
reach for little stars from your mattress.
The blackness
lit up by a flicker of some matches.
Anxious
we'd sit and watch them burn black to ashes.

Ashes to ashes
and then
dust to dust.
We'd talk dreams around the table hoping nothing would
rust.
Just us
little kids wearing pockets of trust
hoping we'd pick up on a dream
that would stick and then last.

I Don't Want To Settle

We were kids around a table, planning a life.
Dad, he lifted his liquor with open mouth in advice.
'You kids have got it now but life it holds like a vice.
So do what you love,
fuck the rest.
You've got time.'

Dan Whitlam

He was at the back of parties
sniffing white off car keys.
Making
two-hour friends with those who popped pills like Smarties.

Making
dinner dates he'd never go on
with them fake Kens and Barbies
thinking a night would never end.
But
they were kicked out
so followed suit to a random kitchen at 4am.

Listened to Maroon 5.
Lost in their balloon highs.
Sniffing lines in hopes to find that feeling of the
first time again.
But
anxiety will probably kick in a minute.
Come with the sunshine and birdsong.

But
you thirst on drinking gin topped with the tonic of nothing
as you realise these aren't friends.

I Don't Want To Settle

No
they're strangers.

And tonight's highs
are just
borrowed happiness from tomorrow.

Dan Whitlam

Growing up means
growing apart.

It means bumping into a childhood friend
you shared sandwiches with but not knowing how
to pick up the memories over coffee.

Growing up means
remembering to drink water every day.

It means having a skincare routine,
in high hopes Vitamin c will brighten the darkness from
last year.

Growing up means
buying crockery.

Matching plates and bowls that you bring out
at cook clubs and dinner dates
inevitably to be dropped or chipped by so-and-so as
the third bottle of Beaujolais spills over.

Growing up means
run clubs. Baking banana bread.
Long weekends and cheese.

I Don't Want To Settle

All the cheese.
Despite being told you are lactose intolerant by various
healthcare professionals.
Taking the short-term win only to suffer
the consequences the next day.

Growing up means
figuring it out.

Discovering what you love and how you
want to live this life of yours.

And growing up means
finding a person you want to share it all with.

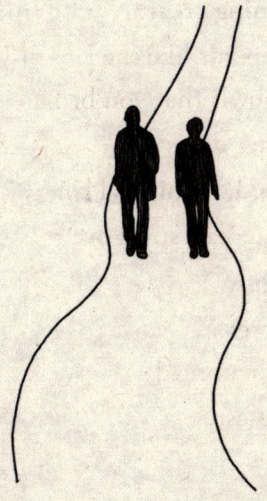

Dan Whitlam

 She wore baggy hoodies
with tie-dye Levi jeans.

Saw herself as a problem teen with a head full of dreams.

She was a kid with promise
but
therein she lacked self-esteem.

So
she kept running up that hill with Kate Bush set on loop.
Smoked Kush to feel loose and
swore the arts held truth.

She was a deep sleeper.
Stay in bed not a morning creature with fine features.
Cheek bones were deep-cut like the ribs of Jesus with
eyes of Venus.

Deep pools of blue that left you speechless
but
find a subtle glint within
like her eyes held a secret.

Her name was Nina.

I Don't Want To Settle

And she was a strong believer that
maybe it's okay to not have it all
figured out.

Maybe we do have so much more time
than we think.

Dan Whitlam

 Well, she was down on herself
just wishing she had someone to say:

*Sometimes the sad feels better than feeling good
and that's okay.*

Sometimes we do want blue skies
to fade away into clouds of perfect grey.

She thought
a life of just happiness sounds pretty sad anyway.

She'd tide herself over by tying blankets around her waist
racing around the room with the powers she so craved.

She was superwoman.

A super suit that suited her best.
Red trails flew behind her with an S on her chest.

See
with that blanket on her body she could be anyone.
She could be anywhere.
She could beat down on the sounds of lonely and scared and
break away from the bubble that troubled her cares.

I Don't Want To Settle

It was a path to a new you.
But
who knew that she too would run around with such blues.
Passing people in pain but
she'd just smile on through.

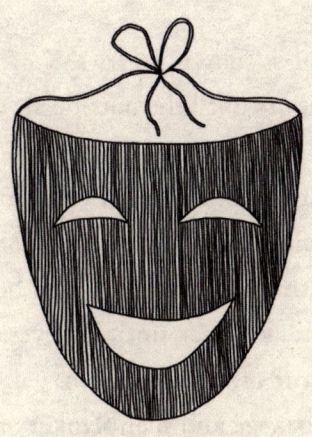

Dan Whitlam

 She wore her grandmother's pearls
and
summer dresses down to her knees.

Drank white wine from the bottle
and always stopped to climb through trees.
She was a wild child: trouble.
Didn't really care to please.

And she'd read.

Often, alone for hours until the outside air would turn ink
black
sending her running back inside for comfort
swaddled in her mink wrap.
Had distinct hair that she plaited in tight holds.
Would listen to Frank Ocean until her eyes slowly closed.
And there she'd drift off into an ocean.
Floating through orange and that blanket of emotion.

Dreamt up thoughts of travelling
in between a nine-to-five.

I Don't Want To Settle

Consumed by the thought
there's more than one way to live this life.

And
it wasn't there to be lived for others.
Just yourself.

Dan Whitlam

There's an incredible comfort
in knowing that loneliness
is one of the most universal feelings.

On the days when
we're not strong enough to hold up ourselves

we're reminded
that the universe forever has our back.

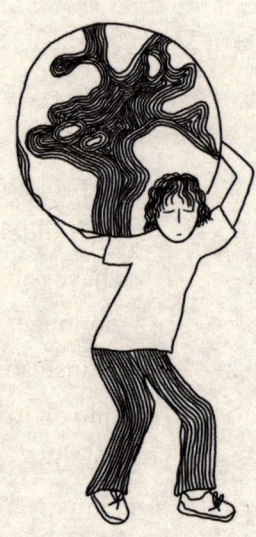

I Don't Want To Settle

I'm fortunate enough to say that I grew up in two other countries before settling down in London.

I lived in St Petersburgh, Russia, and in Istanbul, Turkey. At the age of nine, while trying to coax my mum and dad into admitting they were international spies (surely the only reason for living in both Russia and Turkey?), my older sister Lily suddenly burst into the room in floods of tears. The cause of her upset? She was unsure what she should study at school the following year. 'What should I do at university?' she asked them. 'Why are we living abroad? Why am I here? What should I do with my life?'

In hindsight, these were all very fair questions coming from a 12-year-old. However, at the time, my 9-year-old self couldn't wrap my head around her panic. I didn't yet know the responsibility that comes with decision. Surely you just carry on as you always have? You do next year what you've done this year. We're living here because Mum and Dad took us here, and we'll probably do something similar to what they do when we get older.

My sister seemed to have had a real moment of realisation surrounding choice – no longer just accepting that this was the way things were and instead questioning everything. She was turning the status quo on its head and shaking it all up to see what answers came tumbling out. She wanted to know why she was here but, more importantly, what she should do with her time here.

My mother, who sadly passed away a few years after this conversation took place, gently took my sister onto her lap and told her about a Japanese concept called *ikigai*, which broadly means 'one's reason to live'. Wiping Lily's tears, she told her that *ikigai* consists of finding happiness through four elements:

What you love.

What the world needs.

What you are good at.

What you can get paid for.

It's now generally accepted that this is a Western interpretation of *ikigai*, but it certainly gave my sister some questions to consider at the time. Of course, discovering that one 'thing' or 'skill' or 'job' that appeases all four elements is no easy task. But to have something in your life that does agree with even one or two of these elements is a start. The elements serve as a reminder to do what you want to do, not what someone else wants you to do. We are human, and what you love to do may change over time. And that's completely okay. Change brings growth, and maybe it's the beauty of being exposed to new experiences over time that brings us just as much happiness, rather than finding that one thing you want to spend your life doing.

I was lucky enough to be exposed to performance and the arts on my tiny school stage in Istanbul, playing Mr Mistoffelees in a very tepid rendition of *Cats*. However, so many of us don't have that exposure. It's easy to take these words on the surface, but ultimately things like privilege and environment do come into play. Regardless, everyone deserves to have some time to figure out what they love. To be open to the fact that you might not know what your purpose is, and that your favourite future job might not even exist yet.

Feeling misunderstood or lost is such a strong theme that runs throughout our twenties (and even well into our thirties), but I do think that when my mum took my sister Lily into her arms and spoke to her about purpose and *ikigai*, her main point was that *you have so much time*. You're not running out of it. You don't have to have everything figured out yet. Allow yourself the time and space to be able to look at these four elements and slowly figure out what truly makes you happy, rather than doing something that might make someone else happy.

Or, as Paul Dano's character in *Little Miss Sunshine* puts it: 'Do what you love and fuck the rest.'

If I were able to go back and give a piece of advice to my

little red-headed self, it would be that my mum, *ikigai* and Paul Dano were all correct. We really should be living this life for ourselves, figuring out what we love to do, and then doing exactly that.

I Don't Want To Settle

Today, you're twenty-something.
And too soon you'll be thirty-something and a day

saying you don't want to grow older but
don't want things to stay the same.

You want change to frame your life
as you reach for further stars.

But sometimes to be
still
is to acknowledge that you're perfect
right
    where
        you
            are.

Life of dopamine and Baileys.
Been smoking too much lately.

I'll treat a night out as therapy
just hoping it might save me.

He said, 'The buzz is crazy.
I love it
but Mondays hate me.'

I won't go out but the thought of fun
always
somehow persuades me.

What might await me if I just put my head down and worked?
Simply shifted into first; until I
found enough drive to ride off and continue through till morning?

Threw caution to the wind,
like that breeze of change isn't haunting.
I know a dream is what I want but
struggle to take the steps that are important.

I Don't Want To Settle

I'm feeling lost but the world doesn't like
to see people stalling.
Don't like to see when you're exhausted.
When you're down and you're falling.

I'm feeling lost.

I wish I had a bit more time.

Next to a later summer sun
we sit backed up on a blanket.

Mum's peanut butter sandwiches
clutched close over flowered ceramics.

'Life's a picnic,' you say.
'Amongst empty glasses and bottle stains.'

Through the flame we chew cigars and strip the ash away
dreaming of the words
we wish would smoke into our yesterdays.

And
while ash slowly floats and orange embers stray
over Pinot Noir and Beaujolais

you whisper,

'Darling,
we're but broken things with many a broken thing to say.
We're the downers and the daffodils.
The rose garden next to sleeping pills

we're but
beautiful little things,
until life gets to us.'

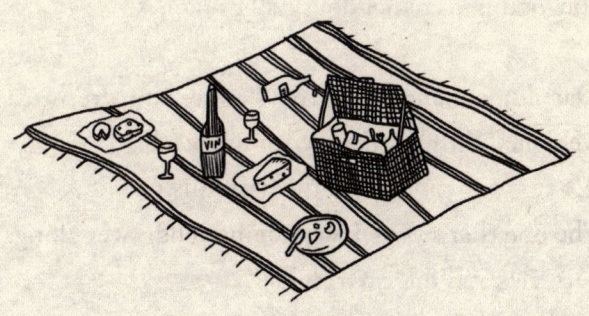

Dan Whitlam

What would you change?

If I could re-live my twenties I wouldn't change a thing.

I wouldn't change the panic years.
The not knowing what to do or where to go.

I wouldn't change the heartbreak.
The first dates in overpriced wine bars comparing how
many brothers or sisters we each had
while attempting to trade gazes.
The first holidays where we'd stay up too late explaining
our dreams to one another
before realising we were living them.
The first fight.
The second one.
The one three years down the line that eventually parted us
for good in a tremendous ball of flames.

I wouldn't change the letter I wrote you afterwards.
The one I didn't send.

The one that sits as a 'what if' in my drawer alongside dead
batteries and ink cartridges
rendered mute by the fact that
some things are better left unsaid.

I Don't Want To Settle

I wouldn't change the friends I let down.
The times I didn't show up because I couldn't make it out the house.
The texts of *I'm ill again.*
I'm running behind
or *I'm hungover.*
The lies I told.

I wouldn't change the truths I told either.
The honesty I shared with friends, family
and myself.
Looking in the mirror and accepting myself for who I am.
Despite the flaws and fights, here you are still standing.

I wouldn't change the wasted time.
The hours spent figuring out what I love and I like.
The hobbies.
The cookbooks.
The gym classes.
The roommates.
All tried and tested, like dipping a pinky in the pool to figure out what temperature fits you best.

Dan Whitlam

The New Year's resolutions that lasted two weeks.
The broken promises.
The ones you learnt from.
Forgiveness. The way you forgave yourself.
The way you forgave them.
The time you didn't.

I wouldn't change any of the beauty I experienced.
I wouldn't change the pain I felt either.
Maybe your twenties are for feeling it all and
falling for it all too.

Falling for it all in hopes you can tread with more
confidence
when
you finally decide to get back up again.

I Don't Want To Settle

He was feeling down and worthless.
Constantly nervous.
So
stayed in bed staring at the ceiling
while questioning what's his purpose.

Living hurt him still.
And so he would stay in his room
just dreading the day

replaying the same phase of closing the curtain until
the sun sank and slowly passed away.

And there he fell a little deeper.
A little bleaker.
A little closer to the Grim Reaper.
Hoping a deep sleep would take the worst of it and
rid him of this fever.

But
really
he just wanted someone to ask him if he was okay.

Dan Whitlam

 She'd always sit on the same train to work.

Plagued by the words
of feeling like
she was running out of time.

A line she'd heard
but never really learnt to listen to.
Didn't make the decision to.
Instead spent her days replaying the same phrase of
how she's missed her youth.

Worked a job she hated
and
that job dictated
the way she'd live her life.
But
never really thought to stop and change it.

Knew she couldn't sustain it
this vicious cycle of hers
where each day felt the same.
Each day waking up to the same alarm saying:

'Yes, darling, go and try again.'

I Don't Want To Settle

The pain of it all was that she couldn't speak to her friends
as they seemed to smile with age

had jobs they liked, relationships they loved
or a faith it would come at some stage.

And so she'd sit on the train
with all these thoughts clouding an anxious mind.
Wondering
Is this what life feels like?
Why isn't my train running on time?

Until she saw it. One morning.
Through the softness of morning eyes and tepid coffee.
A poster of a young girl running from a grey cloud
out and towards the open air.

Shouting and screaming, 'Darling, slow down.
You're doing fine.
You can't be everything you want to be before your time.'
And,
'There's so much time left before you.

So please don't wish it away
by wishing you had more.'

Dan Whitlam

I'm missing days upon the playground.
Paper planes that we threw on through the grey clouds.

We'd pray for rain hoping
clouds would slowly break and
fill us with the feeling of a future as it came down.

I miss the faint sound of *I can't wait to be grown*.
Wishing away our childhood
while getting wet to the bone.

We'd play mums and dads and getting married
in hopes one day we'd have one of our own.

Not knowing that when we grew up
we'd wish that time was suddenly slow.

We'd wish to go back to back then.
Back to playgrounds and fountain pens.

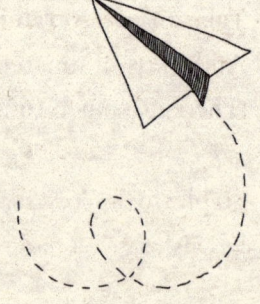

I Don't Want To Settle

Sit in the kitchen, listen to Radio 4
and gaze out the door
a little vacant and bored.

The pain stays like a stain on the floor
so I hedge my bets for a second and then I set off for a walk.

I call my dad and say, 'I'm bored of all the same advice.'
Same dreams that we find under fading lights.

I want a future a little crisper than the bacon bite.
Reaching higher heights than eyes
searching for straying kites.

Wading right into the question of I could,
I might?
But close my eyes for a second,
too scared to set my sights.

Take a cigarette, and smoke it to the evening light.
And think of nineteen, how I saw it through the dreamer's
eyes.

Dan Whitlam

 I hate that photographs
now tell me all I've lost

rather than all I've had.

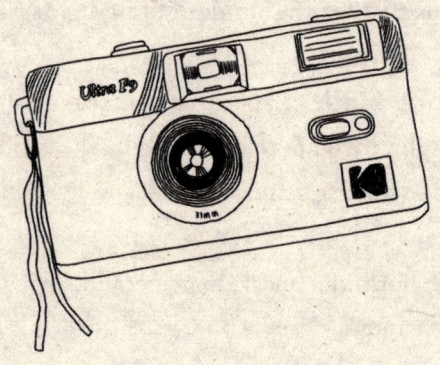

I Don't Want To Settle

Now I can see you on that corner with your stories told.
Nineteen, daydreaming with your Marlboro Golds.

In pouring cold cigarettes you fought to hold
and figure out your future
like your days were turning all to stone.

Writing poems about missing your bed.
Hope to speak it out,
but try and listen instead.

Thoughts upon the paper that you pencilled in lead,
not quite a boy nor a man, yet you act it instead.

Head full of nothing.
You're down and out.
Said it's 'tough' and
you miss your mother so much
you say that you 'suffer from loving'.

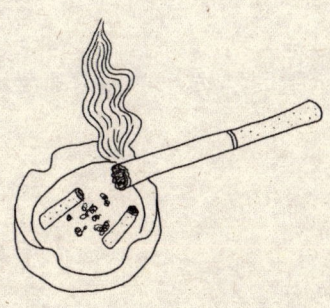

I asked her:

'If you could be one thing in this world
what would it be?'

'Interested
and interesting.

or...

curious
and questioning.

Yeah.

To have a lightness within my eyes
that my soul was reflected in.'

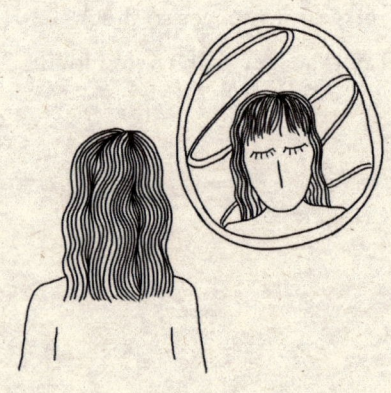

I Don't Want To Settle

This is for those who are
second-guessing and feel the stresses of vocation.

The nine–fives that wear you down
in a world of constant rotation.

If you choose to change your days
and run a different direction
love running where you're going
not crawling in hesitation.

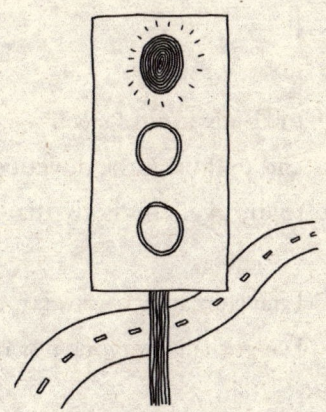

When I was sixteen, I had an altercation with another boy that was very serious and very real. I was left changed by that day forever.

This is the story of that altercation.

It started like any other day. I was sleeping.
And then I woke up.

I

I rub my eyes of sleep
and pull back the duvet cover
to uncover this body that's ready to work and discover.

I have an audition today, and it's my first audition to date.
I've got this nervousness in surplus but I'll keep my head straight.
To be late is out of the question so I
hop out of bed and get myself dressed.

Thinking about this audition ahead…

Edinburgh Fringe Festival.
Twenty days. Twenty performances.
My dream at the hopeful age of sixteen.

I Don't Want To Settle

Now, never been one to dream before as I'd
seen and saw the hardship of men who dare to dream and
dreams come crashing down in cries and roars.
But I took a chance.

So, dressed to impress I opened my front door and left,
chest exhaling these feelings of anxiety but my mind was at
rest,
and as I
walked, I addressed the location request
saw that Islington's Pleasance Theatre was the final
destination of my quest.

I walk to the tube station and
down the wet steps to hear the slurred words
'spare change'
coming from rotten clothing.
There was a beggar on the damp steps, his eyes half-closed.
I supposed he was dozing.
There's a needle in his arm though it's decomposing his
emotion.

But I just kept walking.
And I hated myself for that whole journey, because I could
have stayed and talked,
could have sat with him in the cold. Maybe even gone for

a walk but I, the more fortunate privileged guy, just kept walking.

I arrive at Caledonian Road Tube Station and tap out with my Oyster card.
Sheltering from the rain, I roll a thin cigarette.
Revelling in the feeling of rolling crumbling tobacco between my fingertips.

As I proceed to light and smoke the cigarette, a gang of five hooded men run past me.
Shouting and swearing, passing the phrase
'He's a dead man' to one another.
I watch them run away from the station and around the corner leaving
me in the rain.

I put them out of mind, just five kids messing around.
I close my eyes and allow my mind to be drowned out by the rain's sound.

I focus on my audition.
As I turn the corner, I see a sight that bites at my eyes.

It's a darkening pool of blood surrounded by the hoodies that ran past me a minute earlier.

I Don't Want To Settle

They're stamping on the face of this limp lifeless form,
there was no stop to this beast, no peace at the eye of the storm.
There was no stop to their rage, they did snarl and did transform
into bloodthirsty monsters begotten from hate and scorn.

And I just froze numb to my bone marrow.
Harrowed by this stench of running blood and the visual of five hooded figures
with five different minds
beating down upon this man not once but five times
and these five different men were five times unkind.
Yes, five pairs of eyes but those five pairs were blind.

And then I see it's my friend who's on the floor
who is broken and is bleeding
now my heart's beating
and these feelings of inner demons are seething
I don't believe what I'm seeing
I'm
looking for higher reasons but meanings have left this earth

and I'm moving. I'm running towards my friend and I'm shouting and I'm screaming 'get the fuck off him'.
And all of a sudden, I'm swallowed whole by this beast. This

beast of rage.
Pushed back and forth between its walls like a pummelling cage.
They're throwing fists from the right,
I'm throwing fists from the left,
then I get hit on my right ear and it all suddenly goes deaf.

I hold my head
trying to reduce this cacophony of blows
occasionally lashing out to get them away from me.

I open my tightly shut eyes for an instant, and I see
another figure joining the huddle.
He. Running in from a nearby estate.
As he runs in, I decide I have to move and I have to move now,
so I push off with all my might but I get caught in the crowd
the voices grow loud, I'm caught and I feel drowned
then a hard punch on my back throws me down to the ground.

My head hits the cobbled floor and my nose bursts but
I'm none the wiser
so dazed, I turn over to leave as a survivor
but he stands over me, holding a bloody screwdriver.
We lock eye contact and within those eyes I see a flicker of

I Don't Want To Settle

sadness
like he knows what he's just done
and then he thrusts forward once again, driving the screwdriver
deeper into my right lung.

And then all the voices grow deathly silent, and it's just me alone on the street
surrounded by the echo of my own heartbeat.
I throw my head to the sky and keep my breathing silent soft,
for some reason I still don't know why
I think about my mum.

I think about the words I would say to her since I last saw her.

How I've grown a little older.
And with growing older I've grown a bit bolder.
And now admittedly growing a little bit colder.

II

Well, I rub my eyes of sleep
and pull back the duvet cover
to uncover this body that's ready to work and grow tougher.

Dan Whitlam

I hop out of bed and get myself dressed,
go down the stairs to
leave my house and head on out.

I walk to the tube station and as I get there
I see a guy on the wet steps with a needle sticking out of his veins.
I sit myself down next to him and drop him my spare change.

I tell him about my lifetime, how my mum's going down
a slippery slope, and how I'm doing my best so we can carry on and cope.
I tell him of the darkness in my life, the gentle noose around my throat and
I ask him do we carry on in life or let go and sweetly choke?

And he replied with a few words of peace and happiness,
describing humanity as a lost art form, a museum relic which we once treasured
'Like whatever happened to love thy neighbour.'

He spoke and I listened and on passed time
but after half an hour I had to go
so I thanked him for his mind, I thanked him for his words
of wisdom, and wished him a nice day.

I Don't Want To Settle

But as I walked down those wet steps I
heard him whimper,
'Please stay.'

I hated myself for that whole journey. I could have stayed
and talked.
Could have sat with him in the cold, maybe even gone for a
walk
but I, the guy with whom he saw eye to eye,
kept walking.
I arrive at Caledonian Road Tube Station to go and join my
friends.
North Road Estate where the youngsters take charge.
See me and my friends run a little operation,
a quick intimidation and snatch, rob the other kids so we
can look after our own backs.

But as I leave the station, I bump into my friend Mathew.
And as soon as he sees me he tells me he got a text through
that a couple
kids are leaving the theatre opposite,
asked me if I wanted to roll through for a snatch and grab.
'Nah, man, I'm done with that shit after the chat with
the homeless man I had.'
He said 'Suit yourself' as the five of them walked off,
these five hooded figures with five different minds,

heading off towards the theatre to earn a quick five dimes,
now these five different men were my type of guys
but after just one chat they seemed different through my eyes.

I watch from the window as they run through the courtyard
and on to North Road where the theatre lies.
Running up to and standing in front of the other kids
demanding the pretty pennies in their pockets.
The kids looked scared and dumbfounded and without a word
sounded they handed over their possessions.

But just as one of the kids is passing over his phone
he hits Mathew in the face.

Blood spills from his nose,
now Mathew starts seeing red and they start exchanging blows,
the commotion grows, battle of foes,
blood spread red as a rose,
the other kids now scarper as they couldn't face what they sewed.

I Don't Want To Settle

And Mathew is just
stamping on this boy's face,
again, and again, and again.

It's a sobering sight as the blood begins to darken around
him on the concrete.

I'm thinking they're going to kill him.
He's going to bleed to death,
someone's got to stop this.
Someone's got to stop this.
I've got to stop this.

And so I run,
down the stairs and through the courtyard onto North
Road where the theatre lies,
and just as I turn the corner I see this guy.

Running.
Shouting and screaming, with his heart heavy beating and
his lungs deep breathing,
as he's running towards this gaggle of seething demons,
I know that he's there to save his friend,
to put an end to the bloodshed, to the slaughter put
an end.

But he runs in and with a right fist he knocks Mathew to the floor
and I say, 'No, fuck that, you touch my friend you wage war.'

And I'm running now with adrenaline pumping through my veins
and all the pain in my brain has finally become unchained.
I run over and pull Mathew off the floor, he's got a broken nose and a shattered jaw,
and I go to join the fight but Mathew pulls me back.
He says, 'I don't want him to leave as a survivor' and he reaches into his pocket
and pulls out a screwdriver.

I take it and run on in,
but as I do he sees me and tries to get away,
he gets caught in our crowd,
the voices grow loud,
he's trapped and he feels drowned,
then I stab him hard in the back, which throws him down to the ground.

He turns over and locks eye contact with me.
And within those eyes I see terror, it's haunting me,
it's telling me what I've just done,

I Don't Want To Settle

I can't deal with those eyes.
I stab him again in the right lung.

And then all the voices grow deathly silent
and everyone runs up the street.
I follow close, but all I can hear
is the echo of my heartbeat.

I'm at the top of North Road now and he's at the bottom
lying in a pool of his own blood.
Something inside of me tells me
I have to call an ambulance.

I can't just let this guy bleed out and die,
simply stand by as death sings its sweet lullaby.
We may not have seen eye to eye but I'd be horrified if I just
stood by and
let this innocent guy die.
I pull out my phone from my pocket.

When I was sixteen, I was stabbed twice in the back with a screwdriver in Islington. My lung collapsed and I was rushed to hospital.

Two years later, through a practice called restorative justice, I was able to meet the boy who stabbed me. It was a chance to find out what his story was, why he was there that day and what his motivations were.

Although incredibly traumatic, the stabbing also brought about a lot of realisations for me. Lying in that hospital bed, I found myself thinking about what was truly important to me. After coming so close to losing it, what did I want to do with my life?

Maybe it's in the moments when we're injured or forced to slow down that we really get a chance to think about what we want: to be still, re-evaluate and reflect upon what we've had and therefore what we perhaps want to do differently.

In between the blips of my heart monitor and groans from neighbouring patients, I spoke to my dad about the idea of turning pain or trauma into art. Was it possible to turn a bad episode into something good? For some reason he decided to broach the subject of what I wanted to do at university. *A perfect time for that, Dad*, I thought. But, maybe for him, speaking about the future would brighten this current ugly present? I told him I still didn't know what I wanted to do for certain, but I liked the idea of doing something in the arts. Music. Writing. Something in that field. My *ikigai* perhaps?

The poem you've just read was written during my first year at drama school. My first poem. A very eccentric teacher of mine had asked us to write about something that meant a lot to us. Something that changed us. I decided to write up the account of that day from both sides.

After I finished writing the poem, I felt an enormous sense of peace and clarity. I do think at the heart of the stabbing we were just two young men who were swayed by their emotions. Two young men feeling lost. Myself, running over in the heat of that moment to protect a friend; and him, seeing his friend being hit doing the same. And isn't that a big theme of your young adult life? Being swayed by your emotions and acting out of impulse rather than lived experience, rather than logic or reason?

Before that peace, however, I did spend a lot of time scared to walk around without my dad acting as some sort of chaperone. Taking me to and from the tube station and friends' house parties. I was plagued by anxiety, the stress that it might happen again.

It may seem painfully obvious, but that anxiety and worry only left me after I forgave him. The boy who stabbed me. Only once time had passed and I was able to distance myself from that day, after I was able to write about it, was I able to forgive what had happened. Forgive myself for running over and also forgive him for doing the same.

Such a huge part of your young adult life is making mistakes, so shouldn't a huge part also be about forgiveness – for others, and also for ourselves?

Part II –
You and I

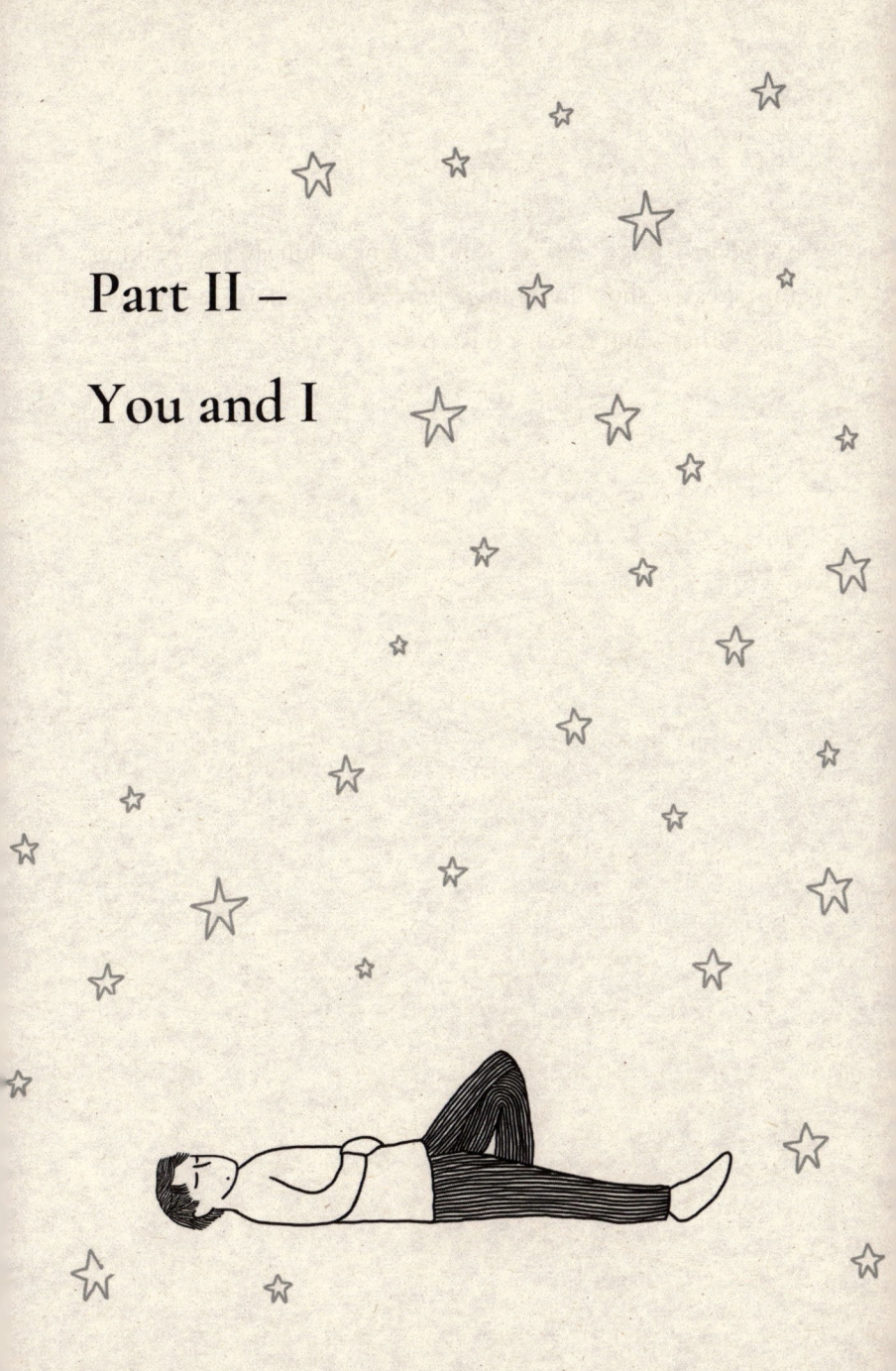

I Don't Want To Settle

I've always been a strong believer that we take a lot from our parents, or the people who raised us. Especially how they were in a relationship. You noticed how they treated each other and cherished the idea of love and partnership.

My dad David, as I mentioned earlier, lost his person when he was just forty-two years old. I asked him many years later if he ever considered looking for someone else, or even re-marrying. I probably asked in a naïve way, as if a choice like that could be made easily.

My dad's response was short and beautiful:

No, never again. She was the love of my life.
The only one I want to remember.

Dan Whitlam

If I had three lives, I'd marry you in two.
And in that other life
that slightly slower
dimmer one
I probably would have been a writer.

Sat up in corner side cafes trying to pen you into existence.
Not knowing you but
still knowing I was missing something.
A part of me that would have made me a little more whole.
A little more together.
And so, I'd write.
Penning the idea of you to paper in hopes you might form
out of ink and our story might begin.
And that's not to say I wouldn't be happy in this life, of
course I would.

I'd have friends to laugh with.
And complain about how much or how little work I'm
getting.
Set in a small apartment overlooking the river
filled with books and faded denim in a desperate attempt to
look far more interesting than I am.
And on the weekends, I'd walk that water.

I Don't Want To Settle

A little slower and a little dimmer. Wondering
if I'd ever meet you.

> My response to 'If I Had Three Lives'
> by Sarah Russell

Dan Whitlam

 I want the type of self-love
where you can look in the mirror and say:

I want to grow old with you.

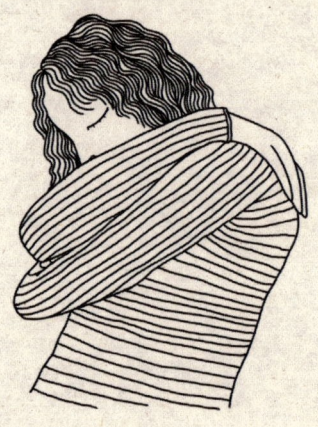

I Don't Want To Settle

Let me pass you a bouquet
of forget-me-nots.
And

as I pass them to you, I whisper:

'Forget me not.
For
people in this life tend to forget me a lot. But
I won't forget what I love and I like and like these forget-
me-nots. Darling,
please don't forget me tonight.'

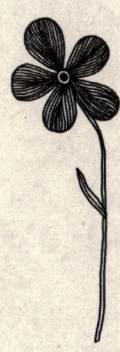

Dan Whitlam

I don't want quick intimacy.
I want someone to lean into me for a lifetime like how I
dreamt it was meant to be.

Holding you through the still days
and then the hurricanes too.
Anyone can do the honeymoon phase but
true romantics hold for the distant moons that are deeper
and blue.

Was told we were supposed to spend our lives with
someone
and that someone would be your journal.
The first person you tell everything to.

Writing in the pages of their spine. Like
the days left to write would last as long as you do.

Maybe I romanticise love? Through old movies and
YouTube. But
the thought of me and you in a house with a view
that's the kind of old movie that I could get used to.

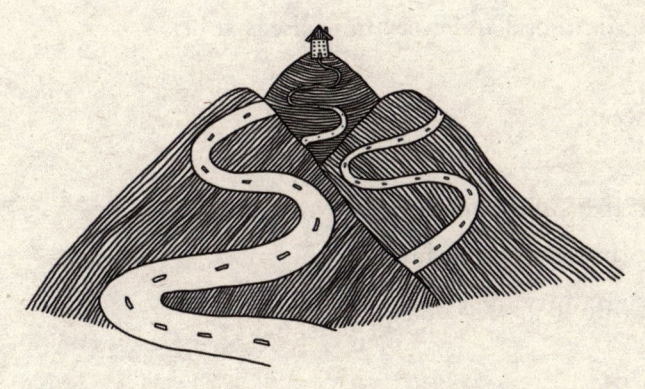

Kiss me so deeply
that I can taste your dreams.

I want to feel the episodes of your life. Where you're headed and where you've been.

The long walks and routines.
Childhood through rude teens. Your growth
into adulthood and everything else that lies

between.

And that's the scene between you and I.
Laid awake in bed, while I

paint infinity signs down your spine.

        Counting the
           goosebumps down
     your back as
they ripple
        up to your
             mind.

Taking my time to outline your finer features. Like my fingers were walking blind.

I Don't Want To Settle

I want to paint you in respect. With colours you won't
forget. And
on days that come darker
they'll take the pain from your silhouette.

So go and rest for a while
as I write love notes down your spine. Written in the silent
hope
I'll still be writing them
in five years' time.

Dan Whitlam

 Take that love
the deep swathes of it that they don't want
and smother yourself with it.

Holding yourself so tightly until you are drowning
in you.

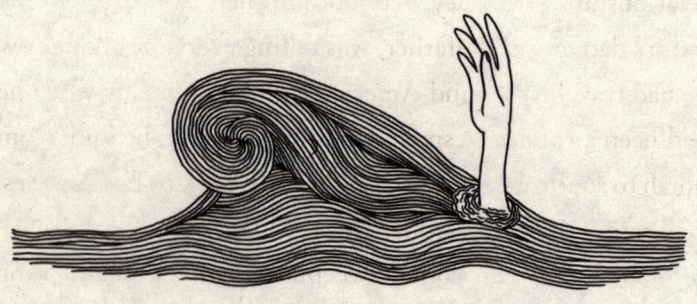

I Don't Want To Settle

While love can be consuming, profound and serious, it can also be very silly.

My dad has Tourette's syndrome, and my sisters and I have inherited parts of that as well. For me, it mainly manifests itself in occasional twitches here and there. Head movements. An eye twitch.

My previous partners always said they found it endearing when I'd accidentally tap them on the shoulder with a head twitch as we cuddled up on the sofa, though I've always been slightly sceptical as to whether this is actually the case.

One of my dad's ticks was singing 'when the wind comes sweeping down the plain' whenever someone said the word 'Oklahoma' (at fourteen, he'd spent four months straight rehearsing for the musical at his school) and once told me a story about the time he was at a family lunch with my mother's parents. This was back in the early stages of their relationship, when they were both in their twenties, and my mum's dad, my grandfather, was telling everyone about how he had travelled around America with his company when he had been a young salesman. He'd been all over, he said, from north to south, east to west – from New York to Los Angeles, Dallas to . . . you guessed it, Tulsa, Oklahoma.

'When the wind comes sweeping down the plain!' sang my dad.

'Your mum loved me despite all my faults,' he would tell me.

It's so easy to get wrapped up in the idea of being or having the perfect partner. With social media constantly showing us a curated highlight reel of seemingly perfect relationships, we are naturally demanding more from ourselves and our significant others.

But do we not all come with an emotional backpack? Our own anxiety and problems that we hope will be accepted by another? Of course we do. But it's the people who love us despite our faults that are the ones we hope will stick around.

Dating in the modern world is hard enough, trying to fit in Hinge dates between gym classes, between overworked anxiety, let alone finding a 'forever partner'.

How can I possibly find enough time for someone else, you wonder, *when I don't even have enough time for myself?*

Often you hear the idea that before you can be in a serious relationship, you need to grow by yourself and become the person you're supposed to be. *I'll work on myself*, we tell ourselves, *and then, I'll be ready for a serious relationship.*

But maybe, if or when the right person comes along, you should be able to grow *with* them – to explore all the wonder life has to offer alongside them.

In my earlier relationships, I often found the worlds of infatuation and love became blurred. Everything was new and exciting and I found our identities became mixed. We became versions of ourselves that we hoped they would like. Saying what we wanted each other to hear rather than what we truly thought. But surely a relationship, or love, is just the meeting point of two people who are operating in their own worlds and happen to want to operate with that other person next to them?

Maybe a lot of growing up is learning how to be yourself with someone, rather than becoming a version of them they'll eventually like?

After hearing that story from my dad, I came to the conclusion that perhaps part of our twenties is about realising what matters in a relationship, about what's important when it comes to love. Discovering that we are not perfect as people, that we all have flaws and that we as individuals have to accept ourselves, in high hopes that a partner will accept us too.

Oklahoma.

Dan Whitlam

 She told me she wished to be a teacher
for education was the key.

'Well, teacher,

you've turned my pupils into pupils
and taught them
better things to see.'

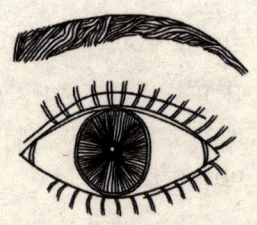

I Don't Want To Settle

Let me bury your hands in soil
until out grows a palm tree.
Your fingers
hanging like fruit
will blow in the breeze and
I'll pick them.

Tasting the places they've been and the wrinkles they've
kept.
For fruit is never sweeter
than when it's eaten
by the one who helped it grow.

You made me
me.
So please
eat from all I have to offer.

For I eat in the silent hope that maybe
I made you
you.

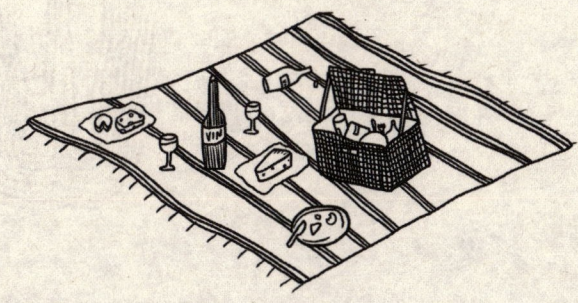

Dan Whitlam

 They have this aura.
This
distinctive atmosphere
that has you ready to give up all your beliefs and morals.

Just to spend a moment
agreeing with theirs.

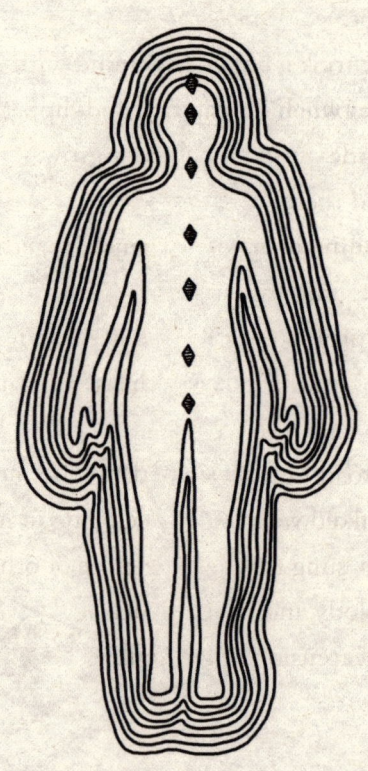

I Don't Want To Settle

We shared headphones through Battersea Park
forwarding songs to their happiest parts
in hopes of sharing little pieces of ourselves.

Our songs.
The ones that move us to our quiet place where
silence is an acquired taste but
damn do we in silence find soul.

She took a hold of my mind with Crosby, Stills & Nash as
soft blue bills splashed and dipped their heads in nearby
ponds.
And there we sat.
Smiling on a nearby bench, together
watching the ripples.
Her soft songs kissed a little and
took my hand down that road of no return.

A road I gladly walked.
Walked with her whole being in my ear.
Yes, sung through the guise of others but, every word,
melody and chord struck
an extension of her soul.

Dan Whitlam

Let our lives be music.
And how wonderful my life is
to have bathed in her symphony
for a little while.

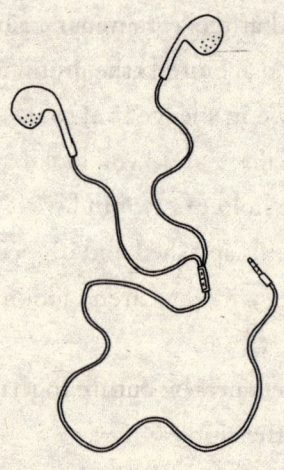

I Don't Want To Settle

It's a brief moment of change.

Like
catching someone's eye on a crowded train.

Staying with them for an instant before
your eyes flash back to the ground.

Taking a pause before you look back again.

And now
you wonder why they aren't looking back too.

You planned a whole future in that pause
in those few seconds
and now you have to watch your future stand up and walk
off the train
never to be seen again.

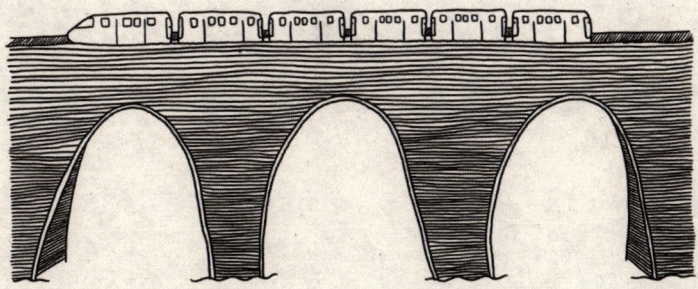

Dan Whitlam

That night we slept above the stars
above the great firmament.

Knowing that not even space
could limit us.

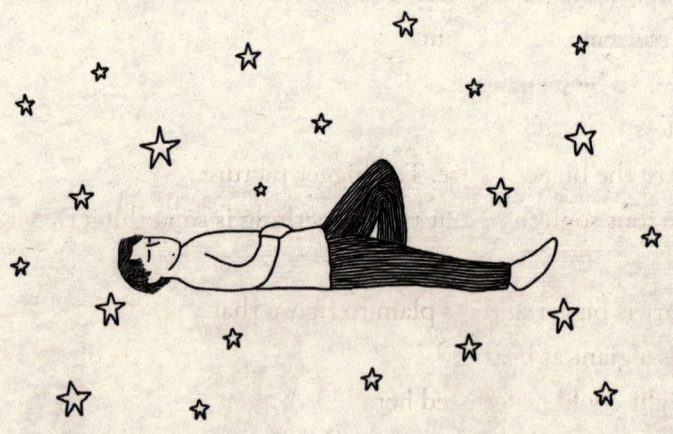

I Don't Want To Settle

To she who takes two steps where I take one.
Whoever thought that
my steps would take your steps to a run.
We stand a foot in height difference
where
just a walk around the block becomes your marathon.

I'll call you Little Big
for, while you might be somewhat smaller in stature
your mind is something I could only dream of measuring up
to.
I love to
hear you speak with the words that form from your mouth.

You skip pebbles across the ripples of my mind for now
but when I'm down in my doubts
you help me figure it out.

I guess
you're the bigger figure. The bigger picture.
Five foot something but that something is something richer.

Heart is bigger and it's plain to figure that
she's a giant at heart.
Height could never need her.

Dan Whitlam

Let me love you like the moon.

Completely with you on all your days,
whether whole, half or barely visible.

Loving you
through every p h a s e.

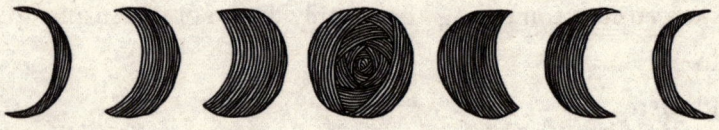

I Don't Want To Settle

Stare into their eyes
like there are stories hidden within.

Each flicker holding a page.

And I guarantee you
the deeper you read

the more you will never want that
story to end.

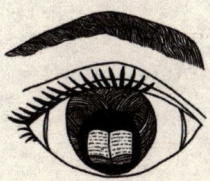
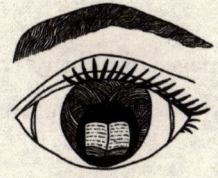

Dan Whitlam

 This is for clothes that smell of each other, scent trailing out of their skin.
This is for those big hoody stealers, dreaming up big thoughts of him.

This is for lips that will kiss her after Sunday rest.
This is for prayers in the church both wearing Sunday best.
I love you more some days and I love you some days less.
This is for honesty in loving, for time is the test.
The ones who stick throughout the shit and all the pits that depress.
The fits of unrest that will a weight on your chest.

This is for no need of speech knowing that looks will do
for there's no need to speak when he's learnt the books of you.
From the pages of light to the chapters of blue.
From your ink-black evenings to your mornings of dew.

I Don't Want To Settle

'A life of love comes with grief,' she said.

'Oh yes,' he replied.
'Always.

But a life without love is a grief not even worth imagining.'

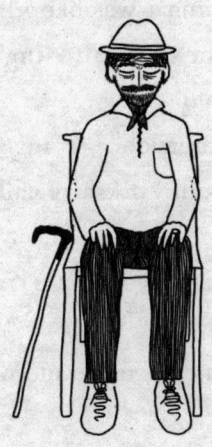 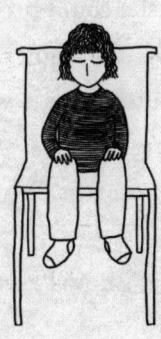

There's something so beautiful about seeing someone's eyes light up when speaking about how they met someone.

I speak about her often at my shows, but my grandma is one of the reasons I got into poetry and writing. We would have long conversations on the phone where she would tell me her stories and I would tell her mine.

She once told me about a time when she was travelling down from Bradford to London on the train and, while drinking a glass of wine, she swallowed her tongue.

Yes. Her TONGUE.

It's a very rare phenomenon, but nonetheless something that can happen. She couldn't breathe, and for some reason, the man next to her knew exactly what was happening. He opened her mouth and pulled her tongue to the correct position so she could breathe again.

Naturally, they got talking after such a strange ordeal. It turned out he was a wrestler from Yorkshire called 'The Masked Kung-Fu'.

Of course he was. What other name would this train hero go by?

'And that's how I met your grandpa,' my grandma said.

What I love about this story is that it goes against here traditional narrative that falling in love is always some kind of perfect, stumbled-upon meet cute. These are the images that we then end up putting ourselves under so much pressure to experience ourselves. In reality, love can find you anywhere – maybe even when you're unexpectedly choking.

It's interesting to think back to a time when you met someone. Was it some grand cinematic moment, or was it just beautifully ordinary?

I don't want to settle.
I want someone to sweep me off my feet and speak it slow that I'm special.

Someone who likes me because but then loves me despite.
Despite all of my baggage, the battle scars and the fights.
I want love that's imperfect.
But, perfectly so.
For people are made from their shortcomings, their worries, their lows.

Know I'll hold you in the same light

through your highs and the downers too.
I'll treat your frowns just like a smile for they're both you.
Both grew from a person, who's split by love and hurting.
We all carry both halves so
I want one who loves me at my worst and accepts me for that. Holds me intact.
Don't want to settle for someone who runs when the going gets bad.
The going can add the deepest meaning to your life.
So
find someone who wants your dark days
just as much as your light.

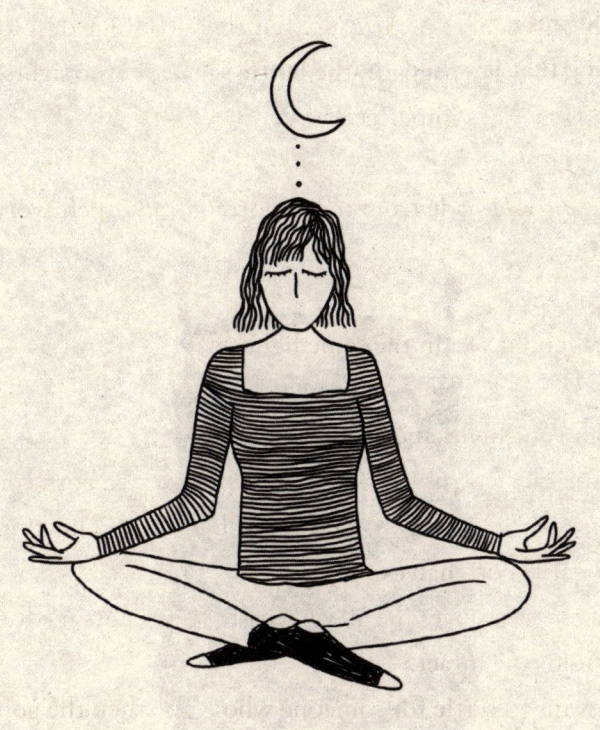

Dan Whitlam

 I miss sharing my life with somebody.
And what a lovely story it would be.

You saying, 'Once upon a time,' and
I would smile
knowing that it would end with me.

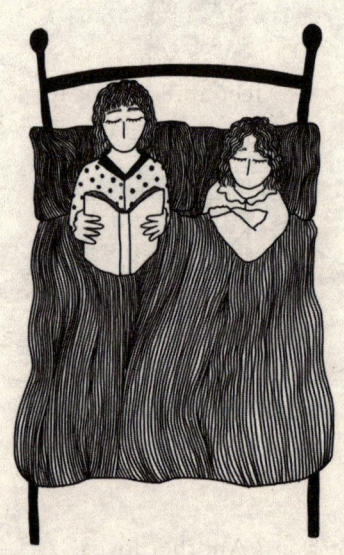

I Don't Want To Settle

Why is it called 'falling in love'?
Why do we fall into this joy?
Falling would surely indicate we are out of control or
rather, engaging in this act helplessly

only to be saved when we reach the end
when we hit the rock bottom of reality as it were.

Is love then perhaps the floor below? The place of safety?
We fall, land
and find a constant.
A safe place to lay our feet and dreams for a while. But
an intermittent one nonetheless.

A temporary floor that keeps us safe before one day we
might
what?
Fall again?
Fall out of love?
Once again plummeting towards
where?
Another floor perhaps? Another love?

A life of falling.

Dan Whitlam

Let us change the narrative then.
Let us rise in love.
Rise through and above all floors that have held us before.
And if it must end
as all great things must
then let us rise out of love too.
With dignity and grace.

Soaring to greater heights that falling
can only dream of.

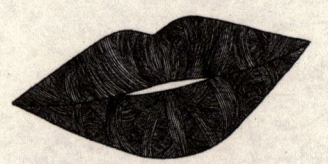

I Don't Want To Settle

We are beings made of stardust.
And
in this moment all I want
is to be the space between your stars.

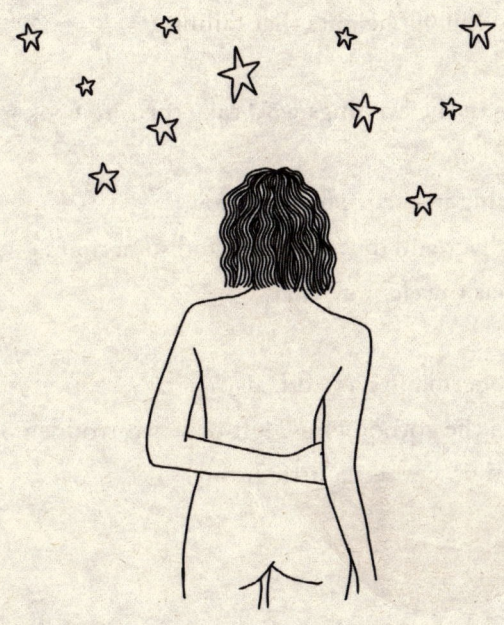

Dan Whitlam

I'd like to think that time has reserved a place for us.
Some simpler time.
Where it did work out
and the world didn't seem so against the idea of you and I.

And maybe in that time we'd find ourselves under a
thatched-roof cottage.
The one you always wanted.
The one we call ours.

And maybe in the evenings we'd take turns to cook for each
other.
Often cooking in silence for we know
that sound lives and dies within it and sometimes
it's wondrous to celebrate that.

Maybe a Dobermann named Daisy
curled up in the corner whose left paw was trodden on
as a pup and now walks a little funny.

I Don't Want To Settle

But
her undying tenacity to still live life to the fullest
serves us a constant reminder that we must play on
with the hand we're dealt.

A time reserved.

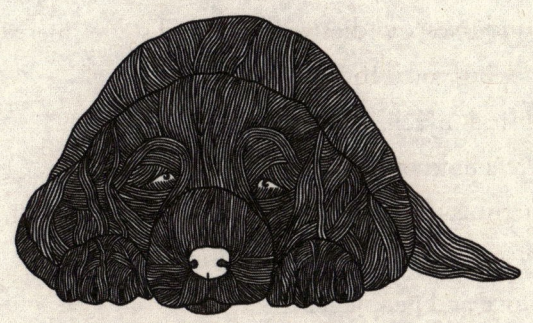

Dan Whitlam

Maybe
it's because you're my person.
The one who holds me together when days seem their worst
and there's nothing better to find.

It's how you slowly remind me that there's more to life
than comparing myself
to those that live it through other eyes.
It's because I feel enough when I'm with you
and life is tough when you've been through
people who walked away with lips
that with love used to kiss you.

So, no – you weren't my first kiss but
here's hoping you'll be my last.
When I find myself in your arms
they take a hold of the past
and quietly say
it's okay
people love and people leave.
Change ruffles at your curtains like an autumnal breeze but
see
that doesn't mean you can't be loved again, my friend.

I Don't Want To Settle

You reminded me that we're never broken forever.
Maybe just a pause in strength.
But as you pour a drink
I pause on the porch to think
and thank the fact that
as one door closed
a glimpse of a window
opened.

Dan Whitlam

 Witness the magic that occurs
when you give someone
just the right amount of love
to let their guard down.

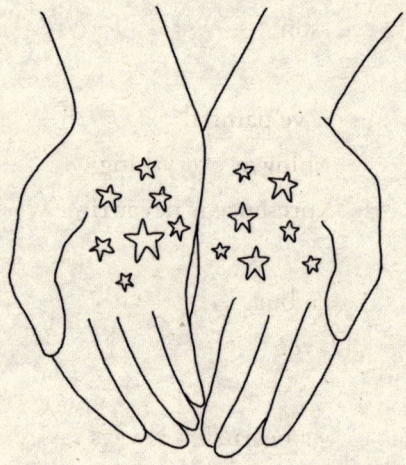

I Don't Want To Settle

We all want to find our person.
The one we wake up and think of.
When we leave sleep
they're the first thing.
The ones who light our life and make us a better version.

They take the grey hours and change them
into something sweet and certain.
Let me find that person

the one in my mind I've painted
the one who sees nothing as everything
even silence in their presence is never time wasted.

It's not stated enough but
what's better than love?

Your counterpart in a heart that always says you're enough.
So
when you find your person
tell them every day.
For they've accepted you for who you are
in your own perfect person way.

A poet talking about love ... shock.

In your twenties, there is so much pressure to find 'the one' – your forever person. These days, we have dating apps that are designed to be deleted and all the messaging we receive – from social media, movies, parents, Valentine's Day – is to find the infamous love that lasts a lifetime. We are surrounded by it. So, when you're single, how else are you supposed to feel apart from thinking 'I should be in a relationship'?

Personally, I'd never want to say that romantic love is necessary in order for us to be happy and complete. Emphatically not.

To be honest, I've had moments where I've been unbelievably happy in romantic relationships, but then also had times where I was deeply unhappy.

I've also been incredibly content, by myself, but then fallen to moments of feeling achingly alone.

When it comes to love, there are so many elements to balance: the love of another person and the love of yourself. Time for your own growth, and time to grow with another. Your own space, and a shared space. Your own hobbies and interests, and the things you love to do together. Dreams of travelling, and the need not to leave a partner.

This balancing act often leads us to examine what our

expectations are when it comes to a relationship. What are your boundaries? Your non-negotiables? Where do you get off or on? Really, it all comes back to how we view ourselves and what we want for our lives.

I've often found that I've loved another person best when I have nurtured an assured sense of self-love. When I've reserved time for myself to be able to decompress from the stresses of work, life, friends, future – whatever it may be – but also dedicated time to pursuing my own passions and hobbies, discovering my likes and dislikes.

After all, if you don't know who you are, how is your partner or a potential partner supposed to know you?

By spending time with yourself and taking care of your own mental health, you get better at setting boundaries. You know what your expectations are in a relationship. What you'll accept and what you won't. What your limits are. You hear about people who are stuck in a relationship or encountering the same problem in multiple relationships, and I've often seen people chasing for things in a partner that they could have found in themselves if they had spent a bit more time looking inward.

Surely, then, self-love and self-discovery are the keys to any successful romantic relationship?

It's important to remember, though, that self-love takes time. It's not an overnight trick that will leave you feeling better in the morning, but a slow, laborious and sometimes uncomfortable process, though one worth doing in my opinion.

In knowing I don't want to settle, I know I need to start with myself if I want to be better in all of the relationships that I have in my life.

Part III – Grief Like the Sky Covered Everything

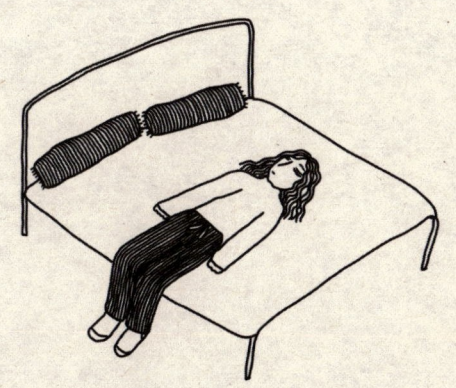

If I could place one book in each and every person's hands, it would be *Tuesdays with Morrie* by Mitch Albom.

It's a delicate story about a young man taking his final university lecture class from a professor who is sadly dying. The title of the class: lessons in how to live.

Albom chose C. S. Lewis's *A Grief Observed* as his favourite book.

After going through a tough breakup a few years back, I decided to pick up Albom's favourite book and was blown away by its honest depictions of grief.

Whether it's a bereavement, a breakup or a shattered dream, grief like the sky covers everything when you are lost.

Of course, the death of a loved one is a completely different grief to that of a breakup. In a breakup, you are left with the strange sensation of mourning a person who is very much alive – having to carry on without them, rendered to imaginings of how they are and what they're doing, asking yourself: *Are they thinking of me? Have they already found love again? Will I ever meet someone who measures up?*

Grief following a breakup is one of the more prevalent forms of loss that I've experienced in my twenties, but when I moved from my home in Turkey to London, I remember being in mourning for my school, my home, my friends – some of whom I haven't seen since. Similarly, there is grief involved when leaving or losing a job, saying goodbye to colleagues, your work place and purpose in order to start again somewhere else.

The natural progression of school life to university to work allows us to meet so many new and interesting people but, in that same vein, we will inevitably lose some of them along the way. As we grow older, our wants and needs change, and those newfound beliefs often don't line up with those we've grown up with and you find yourself parting ways.

Grief brings about suffering; that is an absolute. But what else could it offer? Maybe an opportunity for strength? Resilience and self-growth? After losing my mum, my dad still somehow managed to raise my two sisters and me while maintaining friendships and holding down a job. How he walked through that grief and was able to come out the other end I will never know, but he showed such strength, and maybe that's something that grief can offer?

I Don't Want To Settle

She's married now
and
so am I.
Both very much happy. Very content. Well,
as much as adulthood can make one so.
Both of us fluttering around the soft thoughts of
having children soon.
Starting a family.
'Settling down' as her father would often say after a glass of
Beaujolais or a cigarette.

I do find it funny though, how
years later
when we find ourselves in the same stuffy rooms
at work events or reunions
all those distant yet faintly familiar feelings return.
The old butterflies, re-awoken.
And it's there that I begin to fantasise.
To daydream.
And maybe those dreams will always be.
Maybe
I'll always find the colour of another life in her eyes
as we so gently ask:
'How have you been?'

Dan Whitlam

And, as per the script
we'll both blink and smile
always in polite recognition of what we know to be true.
That it could have been us
settling down.

It could have been us
meeting every morning rather than once every blue moon
in school reunions or stuffy rooms.

Still, we're very happy. Very content.

Well,
as much as adulthood can make one so.

I Don't Want To Settle

 I danced with your ghost last night
listened to Fleetwood Mac as we told rumours in the dark.

Parking ourselves on the sofa
before ripping out each other's hearts.

It was a beautiful death
and I'm glad we didn't pretend.

But, darling
now I've gone and forgotten our beginning
and only remember our
end.

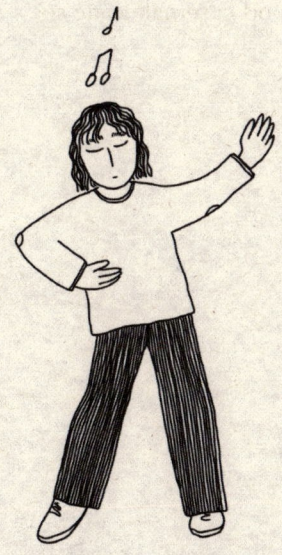

Dan Whitlam

Part of me still believes that you'll turn up at my door
saying,
'Enough of this now,
come over here and let's stop this madness.'
And we'll go back to normal like
nothing has changed, knowing sadly
that everything has.

I Don't Want To Settle

I told myself I wouldn't pick up another pen
until
I'd forgotten the poem
you had written inside of me.

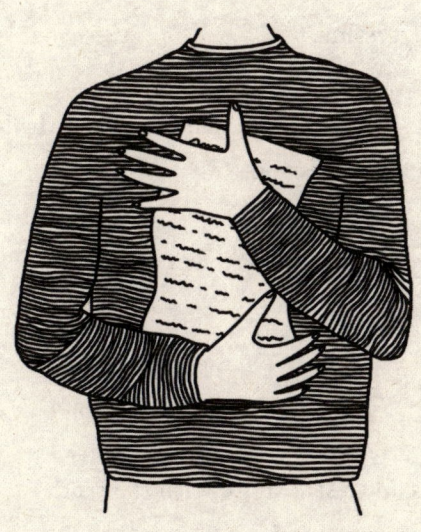

Dan Whitlam

I guess it was a tasteful wedding where
I gave my blessing.
Gold napkins trimmed in pink placed at the table setting.

Green leaves in a glass bowl
that glinted sweet with a maple dressing
and me.

Well, I paced digressing.

Walked towards the bathroom, where I faced the basin
with a blank facial expression.

It would be a waste confessing that I love her,
wouldn't it?

Ruin the best day of her life.
And
my dad always said to stay mute with the truth
if it wouldn't better a mood.

So,
I washed my hands to shake her loose and moved back
towards the room.

I Don't Want To Settle

Watched her dancing for a minute or two, lost in what could have been.
No,
should have been.

Dan Whitlam

How do you count the moments you loved someone
when you have to leave them behind?
No rhyme or reason.
Call it a 'seasonal change'.

We said goodnight without a kiss
before going our separate ways.

But
still the hardest thing to accept in my mind:
how a breeze ruffled at the curtains of change
and told us it was time.

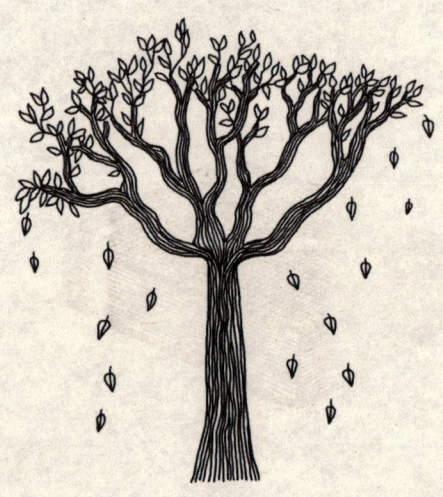

I Don't Want To Settle

My darling was my diary.
The first one I told everything to.
My day-to-days, my dreams and
nightmares too.
But
I guess her pages ran dry.
There's no room for spilt ink.
We closed the book, said goodbye
and
I haven't written since.

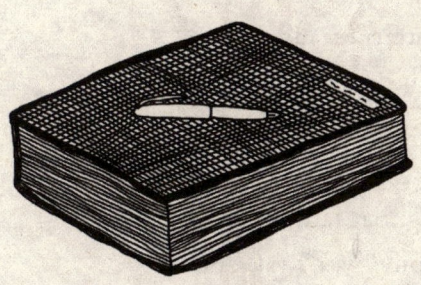

Dan Whitlam

 Placed your picture on the windowsill
in case you walked by again.
I thought it might make it easier
than talking in my defence
but

how does a photo in a frame
hold hope but also change?
I guess I'm caught upon back then
like I'm addicted to the pain.

But still they'll ask 'how are you?'
and like a trick of the brain you'll reply
that you're 'great'
cause you're too tired to explain.

Say you'll 'just be mates'
hoping the bitterness fades.
Same people inside, it's just
we go on separate dates.

Yet, accepting that fate
that's a freedom I won't take. So
I'll live through photos
in hopes
it takes me back to your face.

I Don't Want To Settle

In hindsight
you gave me a single brick
and I tried to build a home out of it.

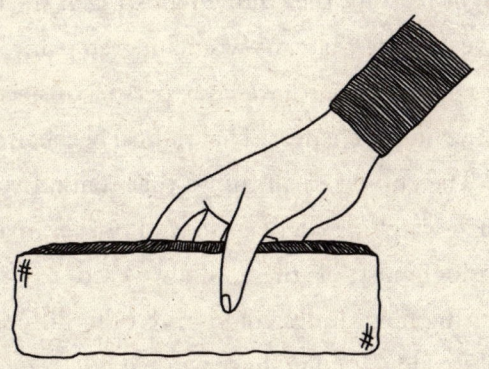

I've been extremely lucky to have had more than one romantic relationship in my life, and each of these has shaped me and made me a better person in its own unique way.

Those relationships eventually came to an end, as all great things must. And as much as I know that each breakup was for the right reasons, they didn't half sting at the time. Most of us have felt it: that gut-wrenching step into the void, knowing you no longer have your person to speak to every day. The inevitable changes. That radical new haircut. Maybe a tattoo? The culling of all things that remind you of them while binge-watching every episode of *Friends* imaginable.

Alongside most of these, I also used to find myself romanticising how things could have been different in that relationship. How it could have worked out.

It's funny that this seems to be the norm for many of us nowadays. We contemplate and question where it could have gone if it went right, even though we're all aware how unhealthy that can be. We wonder if perhaps this is a temporary break, and we'll resume the relationship a few months down the line after taking some time for ourselves. That, this time, the relationship will be stronger than ever and that we'll live happily ever after.

Why do we do this to ourselves?

Is it that we default to this way of thinking in hopes of putting off change? Do we keep writing and re-living the book of that relationship because we fear that if we stop writing, it might die away forever?

In my own personal moments of imagining how a relationship could have been different, it was more often in an attempt to make myself feel less broken. I would return to the safety of memory so I wouldn't have to deal with the all-too-confronting reality of the present.

Dan Whitlam

 I'm forgetting parts of us now.
And maybe rightly so?

Leaving them to the past alongside
first dates and dances
as memory tends to do.

There is a strange sadness in that thought.
Forgetting you.

How someone you painted a soft future with slowly turns
from lover to friend and then from
friend to stranger.
No longer speaking.

But maybe that's the cycle.
How sweet it is to love, lose and then finally forget
all in the blind hope of loving
once more.

And so we do forget.
We leave those we loved most to that darkly lit back room
unstirred.
Alongside first birthdays and the
compliments we're too eager to receive yet too
slow to dish out.

I Don't Want To Settle

It did happen.
So keep it safe but maybe better out of sight?
Out of mind.

Respecting what it served but knowing
that it no longer has to serve you
anymore.

Dan Whitlam

 He was destructive.
Longing for all he'd lost until
he'd lost all he had.

I Don't Want To Settle

 You like to stand in rain.
No one there can see you cry.

Sometimes the darkest skies
comfort the hardest goodbyes.

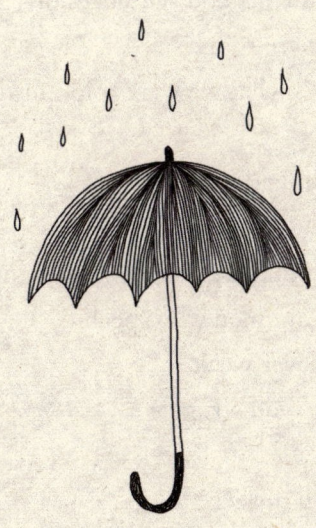

Your life's an upper cut. Toughen up.
Shut it down then button up.
Men were meant for biting down their tongue. Not letting nothing up.
Such is us.
Boys becoming blokes will never soften us. Keep it on the inside
till your problems hide
like sunken
        love.

Nothing but
sentiments and sentences of
'Men are tough'.
That's what we were told but does it comfort much?

Nothing does.

Wish that we could speak it and confront it cos
men are men who speak.
It's never weak
to say you struggle.

Like a dove:
we were meant to fly beyond the sea and mud.

I Don't Want To Settle

But we're stuck.
Stuck inside a silence and it hangs above.
Meaning what?

Meaning we should speak for
men are needing love.
Please. Don't button up.
Open up.
For coping's twice as easy when friends
know how to hold you up.

Dan Whitlam

 How can I even begin to love again
when I'm still so full of yesterday?

I Don't Want To Settle

You loved to read
so you broke my spine and
filled my life with all those pretty pages that you wanted me
to be.

And after you had re-written me
you left me.
Changed and deformed.
Your novel. Half written.
But, in your mind
a better edition
than when you first found it.
People are the pages they surround themselves with, and
I let you muddle the ink in every chapter until
I barely remembered my own name.

Dan Whitlam

 I realise now how selfish it is to assume someone
is in the same headspace as you during a period of grief.
Grief by nature is a solitary and personal response.
I, perhaps, was throwing my own personal mess
on to you in hopes of holding hands through our grief.

But the thing about grief is
there's nothing much to do but march through it.
Alone.
Taking on the pain and hardship, however long it takes.
To do it together would prolong that march.

One of the strangest experiences that comes with a breakup
is
not being able to properly check in with one another
and therefore not being able to properly gauge
where the other person is at.
To know if they are feeling similar sorrow to you.

It's one of the agonies of treating each other like a journal
for the past three years
and then sadly running out of paper.
We can no longer see how each other's days have been
written up.
The highs
the lows

I Don't Want To Settle

the filling meals and
thoughts in between, and so we are forced into imagination.
I realise this is the aim of a breakup.
To slowly render the other person into a figment
of your mind. Or the back of your mind. Remembering the memory of them
rather than specific episodes themselves.

Only our imaginings left to tell us how they are or
what they've been up to.
A coping mechanism I suppose.

But in every single one of these imaginings
I always send you immense waves of happiness and love.

I hope you are doing well.
I hope you are happy.

Dan Whitlam

 He was never one to kiss and tell
threw his lips down the wishing well
and watched them skip into oblivion

with the lips of her as well.

The curtain fell to dead an act that
never really ran its course.
Oh, they'll speak the sweets of marriage but
never the bitter sweet of remorse.

Of course he held his hands up too.
'Was probably me more than you.'

Right person wrong time.
Star-crossed lovers never to collide.

If they wanted to, they would.
It's not you, it's me.
I'll run through every phrase until I find one to believe.

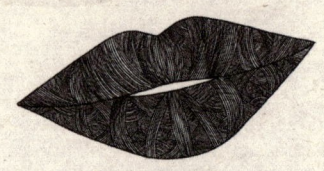

I Don't Want To Settle

'You won't be coming back.'
It took me just seconds to say those five words.
But
years to fully hear them.

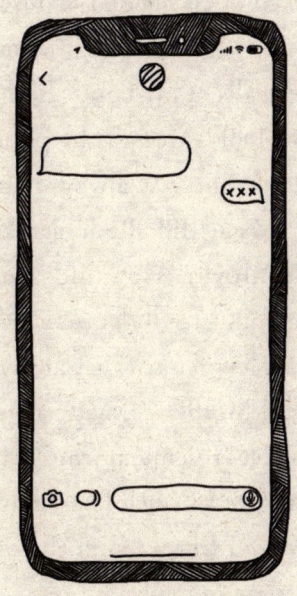

One of the main things about my mum Hannah, besides having a palindrome for a name, was that she loved to take photographs.

Wherever we were, whatever day it was, whether it was a special occasion or not, she would be there, snapping away on her silver Pentax camera. All of these photos she would meticulously stick into albums, hundreds of them, all of which are now stacked up at my dad's house.

It's a wonderful image to think about: all of these memories lining the walls of my family home.

However, when I look through the photos, I realise she was hardly ever *in* any. She was always behind the lens. So when I ask myself, 'What did she look like? How did she smile? How did she frown? How did she sit?', I actually have very little to go on.

Of course, I have a few photos that always circulate when it comes to an annual Mother's Day post on Instagram or a family meal that involves too much white wine, but there are very few photos that give a sense of her character.

I've always wondered who was on the other side of that camera. Who was my mum really?

In a strange way, I've created a sense of her from the way she *took* the photos. Does that make sense? How she would centre certain people. How her finger might be touching the lens, blurring out a tree in the foreground. How my sisters Sarah and Lily smile adoringly at *her* instead of the camera.

And so this poses the question in my head: Is it that *to love* is more than just appreciating the person in front of you, but also how that person sees the world? Appreciating where they find beauty and where they find pain? Accepting them for not just the person you see in front of you but also every other version of themselves? Accepting their past, inner child self as well as their present self?

For is it not everything that we've gone through that makes up the person that we are today?

Maybe to understand how a person sees the world, we need to have empathy for how they have lived it up until this moment? What struggles and victories formed them.

I'm grateful that, as I've got older, I've been able to speak to her friends about her, to understand more about what she was like, who she was as a person.

And so as I get older and gain more understanding about my mum, my perception of her changes. Now, she is no longer just my incredible mother, who would sing me to sleep and turn on my nightlight when I was six years old.

She's also Hannah, the red-haired language genius from Colchester, who met my father by chance in a lift in Bradford and awkwardly asked him for coffee.

She's the young lady who would insist on dancing on her chair whenever ABBA's 'Waterloo' would come on.

She's the little girl whose nostrils would flare when lying about who ate the last chocolate biscuit.

She was someone with a great sense of humour. Who laughed. Who drew. Who fell in love. Who fell out of love. Who felt grief. Who lived.

In essence, she was a human being as vibrant and well-rounded as you or I. Which leaves me with the question, does the way we perceive people and our idea of them change as we get older? Has it for you? It certainly has for me.

There is no doubt that losing my mum and not being able to meet those sides of her as an adult has brought about a slow-burning grief. But I've also found that grief has served as a creative force. I've channelled that longing and feeling of loss into my writing.

Similarly, when I've gone through a breakup, I've found myself at those moments when I feel lowest searching for poetry and words to be able to make sense of what I'm going through.

So many of my songs and my poetry have been written during moments of loss. I've always found that it has allowed me to express myself fully in those moments. Voice what I didn't have the clarity to think out.

I Don't Want To Settle

It would be ignorant of me to say that
I've 'remembered' my mother over the years.

I haven't.

Rather, like a pinky in the pool
she's dipped into my life from time to time. Before
deciding it was better to perhaps not submerge herself into
me just yet.
Better to wait until I'm a little warmer.
A little more receptive to her embrace.
That's not to say I wouldn't gladly swim amongst the
moments and memories of her.
No, I would douse myself in her smiles if it meant I could
take her with me
but the journey I'm on
doesn't allow your best bits with the baggage.

No, they're stopped at the gate and taken out.
Nostalgia alongside narcotics.
Traded for dated photographs, videos and stories from my
father.

That autumn evening in Vienna when she lost her right
shoe and
had to be piggy-backed down the Danube.

And that's where I so wish I could remember the acute details of her.
Her and so many others that I've left behind.
More so to know they actually existed. That what we had was real.
That they were real,
rather than some fever dream after
too much sun in a French July.
The change of it all
at the speed of a butterfly's wings
leaves me dizzier by the day.
Leaving someone behind and marching on without them.
I'm not sure my mind is ready to handle that just yet.

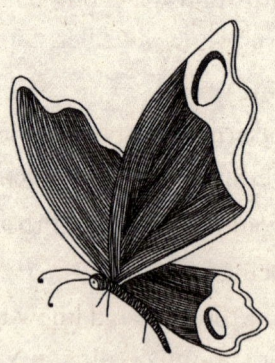

I Don't Want To Settle

In another life I think we might have worked out.

A more forgiving and softer one.

As I pass your perfume on a stranger
I'm not taken back to a painful memory
but back to us.
To what we are. Together.

A softer life, where
we'd sip coffee on Sunday mornings, sat by the fire,
taking in the sweeter notes of the morning grind
before going about our day.

Maybe
hazily walking hand in hand
by the riverbank,
letting time
stand still for a moment before returning indoors.
And this life wouldn't be perfect.
It would still be full of the highs and lows
of being human
but at the end we'd know that we'd still have each other.
That it would work out.

And every day, as you went to put on that same scent
that I've grown accustomed to
that
perfume that would scent the room

I'd think how nice life is now that you've come to sweeten it.

But for now
I'll have to pass a stranger wearing the sweetness of that other life
only to remember the memory.

I Don't Want To Settle

How am I supposed to love you
when I miss the person I met?

Dan Whitlam

 The saddest part about losing someone
is knowing that one day

you'll both
be able to love again.

I Don't Want To Settle

 My whole world stopped
and as I looked out of the window and,
was saddened

that the world hadn't stopped with me.

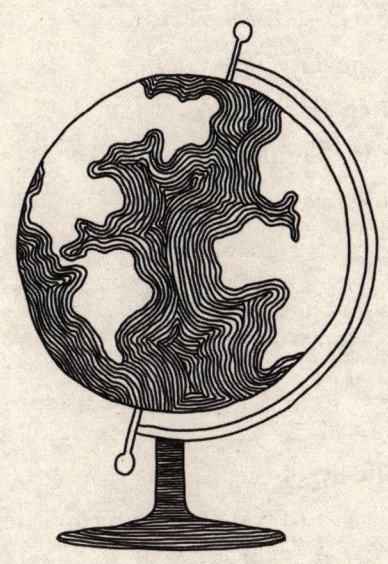

Dan Whitlam

Spoke with rainy eyes,
the boy he hates goodbyes.
Sat by coffins
his coughing to cover how he's cried.
White shirt, pressed.
And his dad's burgundy tie. His shoes, a little big, brogues
fitting double-sized.
Now his worries lie deeper than his feet on the earth.
Six feet.
Dad's deeper now he's off the hearse.
Slowly worsens the day
he heads to church and he prays.
Collect the urn as you turn the corner.
You hold him and say:

'Oh, it's a long life lived,
but sometime it's got to end. So we sing and we drink,
and spare a thought for fallen friends.

Oh, it's a long life lived,
but sometime it's got to end. So we sing and we drink,
and spare a thought for fallen friends.'

I Don't Want To Settle

I don't know if we can be friends.
Not like you imagined anyway.
Cos

that would mean writing over what we were.
All those rose-tinted days.
And
turning it into something less special
and slightly more mundane.

A lower level of pain
where you no longer want me as your lover but
want to hold on to my best bits
while your chest hits the arms of another.

I don't think we can be friends.

But then everyone says it will get better with time
a cruel irony cos
the thing about time is
it takes time.

Dan Whitlam

What do you do with those minutes, months, weeks, years?
Live in a daze without your person
as your days worsen with fear.

You'll close the curtains, as hurting circles then settles and worsens
and now your friendship
is an offer that I'm too deaf to even hear.

I don't want to be your friend.
I just want to go back to back then.

I Don't Want To Settle

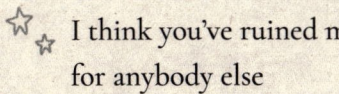
I think you've ruined me
for anybody else

and
I'm okay with that.

Maybe this way
a part of you will remain with me forever.

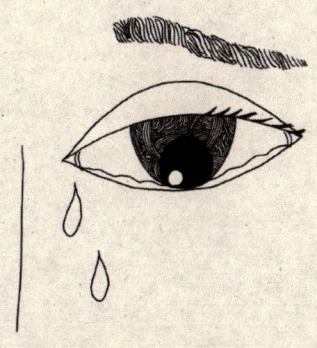

Dan Whitlam

The gift of life is heaven
and here I am screaming into my pillow with the devil by my side
singing me to sleep.

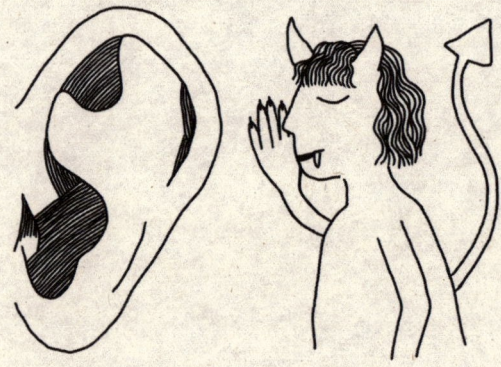

I Don't Want To Settle

Every evening
I would listen to her absence.

Searching for any tremor of life
that might have been left in the dark corners of
our little room.
And every evening
I was saddened that
my mind, often found daydreaming, would still
romanticise our future together.

The reunion.
The tearful questioning and new promises
of how it would be different this time around. Better this
time.

The nervous first evenings.
Re-learning each other's bodies and preferences. The
changes.
Internal questions of, 'Where was that learnt?'
Or, 'Who else has been here?'

The acceptance.
Knowing that progress only grows in the field of change.
Laughter. Children.
Old age.
All found, yet all imagined. But still
I dream in hopes that one day
I'll hear a little knock at my door and smile
knowing that it's you.

Part IV – Look At You Healing

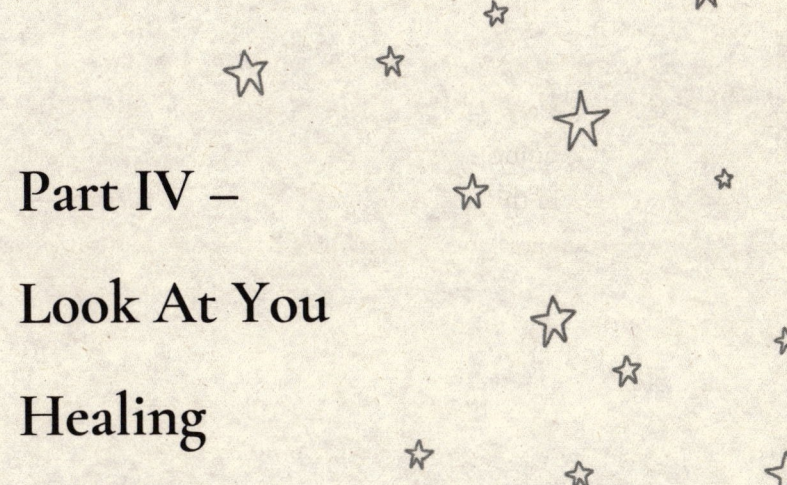
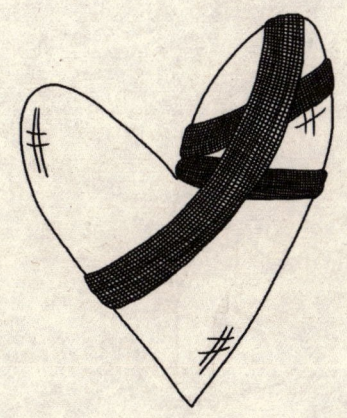

Growing up, one of my favourite musicals and films was *Billy Elliot*. I loved it.

For anyone who may not have seen it, it's about a young boy who also lost his mum at a young age and finds a lot of solace and peace in ballet dancing.

Now, I'm not here to tell you about my thwarted dreams of becoming a ballet dancer, but to tell you about a certain similarity. Towards the end of the musical, Billy finds a note from his mum telling him all the things he should do in order to live a happy and fruitful life. According to my father and my neighbours, my mum also left my sisters and me a note before she died.

Like in the film, it's a note on healing and on living a happy life. Currently, I am yet to find said note, but I will forever keep searching the many drawers of my dad's house to find it.

This next poem was written during COVID, when, like many people, my little sister was going through quite a tough time mentally. In it, I imagined what it would be like to find that letter from our mum, and what words of happiness and healing she might have had for my sister.

Dan Whitlam

 She said in the chapters of life
pain will always hold a page.

And
sometimes the process of progress is
an uncomfortable phase.
But
once you read through the writing you'll see that
lighter days are just a chapter away.
While you're in the middle of it all
don't pretend to be okay.
Sometimes the sad feels better than feeling good so
let it stay.
Let it stay while you spend a smile with a friend.
The ones who hold you in their home without charging you
rent.
The ones who know that you're alone from the way you
pick up the phone.
That lower tone that you own,
they hear it.
They're heavenly sent.
How often do we neglect the down days and spin them with
a smile?
If only we spoke for a while
we'd see that beings are wild and that
feelings like seasons will go and change with the times.

I Don't Want To Settle

So
love all of you
including the sad parts of your mind.

Dan Whitlam

Dear old me,
we're doing a little better now

seen our darker days switch the light on
and our problems
we figured them out.
I'm proud of us today.
Even though we found it hard, we still pushed back and carried on.
Dug our feet in once more
and to the mirror said
'We're not done.'

Despite it all we'll still run.
If we're alive and we're breathing then we must be someone.
And now we wake up a little earlier, without the burning in mind.

I know you feel a burden right now but trust me
we'll learn it in time.

That there's a patience with problems.
It takes some work to beat the fear.
So take a pause and a breath.
You're more than a year.

I Don't Want To Settle

You're more than a moment.

So know that it shouldn't define you.
Just because it's not happening right now
doesn't mean there are heights you won't climb to.
So try to live for today
and live for tomorrow when it comes.

From you to yourself
yourself
who is someone.

Dan Whitlam

 'I'll work on myself
when everything else in my life
is taken care of.'

Work on yourself,
and everything else in your life
will be taken care of.

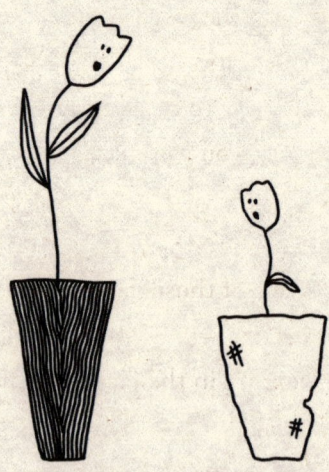

I Don't Want To Settle

I am because you were.
And even though you're long gone they say I still carry parts of her.

That smile she'd often make that would softly crinkle up her nose
or how her eyes would light up at first flowers when spring starts to show.
I know it's easy to think we forget them after they have to go
but, I am because you were and that means
we're forever warmed by their afterglow.

I'll find you in the confidence I hold daily,
in the little lessons you taught.
I find you in the words that I speak and the space of my kinder thoughts.
You taught me to be a better person
even though you weren't here long enough to see me become one.

In the space of those darker days when I'm missing you the most
I take comfort in the fact that I'm here because of you. And for me
that's enough to stay afloat.

Dan Whitlam

 Don't rely on a relationship to make you feel complete

if that person leaves then the cycle repeats.

We keep looking for someone, just continually feed
until you find yourself with another
who can fill what you need
like a temporary glue.

But
what if the missing piece that you seek has always been
inside of you?

Just a little tired and out of sight. But
as it tries to find the light
you fill its shape with different people, hoping this one will
survive.

You should be okay on your own, stop saying it's not meant
to be.
Stop trading problems for people.
You don't need relationships,
you need therapy

so you can steadily find yourself as not a half but a whole.
A whole being
a whole person
who can sit alone with their soul
and feel the world in perfect balance.

So
when you find your person, you'll both live on the same plain.
Two complete people
whose puzzle pieces have found their right way.
Right way home.

Dan Whitlam

I want you to love me
but
tell me how you love yourself first?

How you hold yourself through the hurricanes
when greyer days seem their worst.
Or how you celebrate your little wins
your little things on this little earth.

I want you to ask me about my day
but first
tell me about yours.

Tell me how you sat in silence for sixty seconds
to find a lesson in your own words.

A smaller moment of reflection
self-love for sixty seconds.
How coffee in bed was more
than just a cup from French pressing.

I Don't Want To Settle

Tell me

how you love yourself in a relationship.
Or how you love yourself when you're single.
How do you lean into what you love
until your eyes find a twinkle?
I want you to grow old with yourself
alongside smile lines and wrinkles.

And I hope you want that too.
Cos
everything you love about yourself
is what I love best about you.

Dan Whitlam

 Dear women of our lifetime
you women are our lifeline.
The ones who bring us into this world
and teach us kindness from a bright mind.

The ones who despite it all
are still planting seeds in this ugly world.
Turning fields of greed into fields of green
and hate into lovely words.

And that's mothers and sisters, girlfriends to lovers
the ones who smother us in hugs
when we're downtrodden by what's above us.

The ones who pushed past adversity and still they're
standing with that weight.
The women who had to wait to be seen
cos change in the world was running late.

We need to be better for our women.
More respect for our women.
With your best breath
tell them you love them
for tomorrow is not a given.

I Don't Want To Settle

I want to rise for our women
move with the times for our women.

For women are the ones with wonder that's kept in their vision.

Look. I pray that I listen.
Cos
she spoke and held the whole universe
      between
            her lips.

Dan Whitlam

 You've found your smile again.
The brighter side of yourself you used to only spend on friends
but now you see it everywhere

in every place that you go.
Even evenings by yourself you still feel it when you're at home.

You've found yourself this year.
So
be proud of how much you've achieved.

You used to close the curtain until the sun sank
and only found yourself in sleep.
Better to find your smile in your dreams.
But now you've picked yourself up
and doing better than you've ever been.

I Don't Want To Settle

You found your smile again.
In the mirror on Sunday mornings.
In the little moments that make up the big ones.
No longer a person who's stalling.
You took a step and walked forward. Found a future and ran to it
saying this is my new calling.
So
be proud of what you've done.
As somewhere in the past is a previous you
asking:

'What else is to come?'

Dan Whitlam

 Love will tear you apart. It will break you down.
It will destroy you.

Yes. But
it is also the only thing
that will put you back together again.

I Don't Want To Settle

Happiness isn't the absence of sadness.
It's the acceptance of it.

The knowledge that we are beings of both halves.
Both ups and downs.
And without the two
we would flatline.

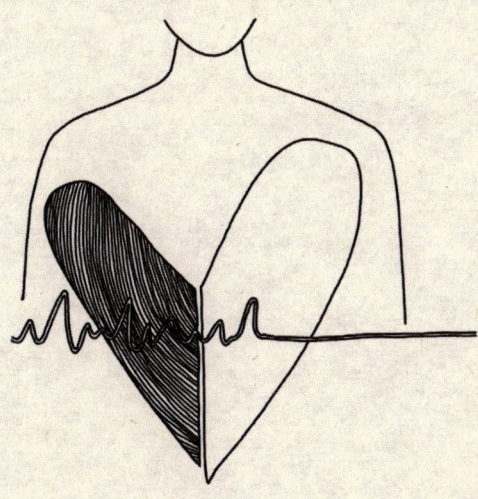

Dan Whitlam

 Held inside her
was an unimaginable brightness

which she never shared
for she was scared how it would be defined.

But, in life
if you worry about blinding a few
the many
may never get to see how bright you can shine.

I Don't Want To Settle

 I didn't listen to that
awful pang in the pit of my stomach on the way home from
dinner that evening.
That familiar tremor of anxiety that has plagued me for so
many years.
The one that told me passersby were judging. Or staring.
Making observations on what I am or more so
what I am not.
I put those feelings to bed.
Left behind with the empty glasses at that dive bar.
The one with the three men in slim-fitting suits discussing
whose Christmas bonus might be bigger.

I didn't listen to my anxieties then either.
When I heard the staggeringly large numbers.
A younger version of myself might have glazed over in the
eyes and
started making quick sums comparing how many shifts I'd
have to pull over the
course of a year in order to get anywhere near to that figure.
Instead I thought of myself yesterday.
Or myself this morning.
Where I was then and where I am now.
How much fuller do I feel?
How much more here can I be?
Remembering that these men too have their own anxieties

their own worries and disparaging thoughts
that keep them up at night.
And so, who am I
to compare myself to anyone other
than the person I was yesterday?

I Don't Want To Settle

She looked me deep in my eyes and told me that the bea
of life
is that even in moments when we aren't present with
someone we love
we're always with them.
We're always there.

Found in the smile lines of friendly laughter that only
siblings share.
Found in the tears that we cry when tomorrow seems cold
and bare.
Found in the blue Decembers when we aren't together.

Remember.
Family lives happy in your heart.
Always there.

with noise in order to avoid the silence

e silence do we find
alisation.

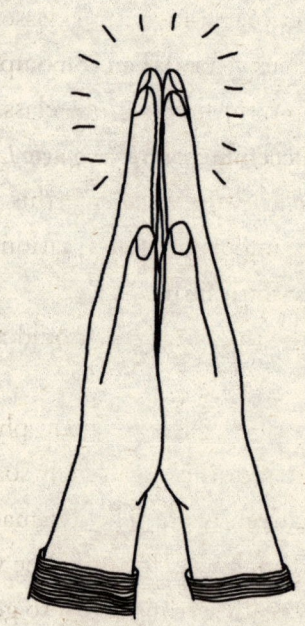

I have a very dear friend who, for the purposes of this anecdote, I'll call L.

Now, L is a wonderfully perceptive and astute man, especially when it comes to understanding how the world, but more so how people, work. I met him in an acting class in London when I was eighteen years old, and am fortunate enough to have called him a friend ever since.

One evening, after one of his acting classes, I was beating myself up about not being good enough compared to so-and-so, not measuring up to my peers in the class. *Why aren't I as good as them? How did he/she create that magic I just watched? I'll never be able to do that.* After vocalising this to L, he sat me down and had a very important conversation with me about the world of comparison.

'Comparison is the thief of joy,' L would always say. And how true that is.

All you have to do is pick up your phone and scroll through Instagram to see others seemingly soaring above and beyond where you currently are. The self-made millionaires, the dream job or dream house, Joe no-name with his perfect hairline and Turkey teeth settling down to get married.

So you think, *Okay, because I'm not there, I must be a failure. I must be wrong.* And we berate ourselves until, more often than not, we give up. We compare until we crash.

We are constantly faced with what we are not instead of what we could be, and this drains us of our happiness and our brightness. What we could be is filled with possibility and wonder and excitement, but in the world of comparison we just think about what we don't have and why we don't have it.

And usually, the things that we *think* we should have, that we berate ourselves for not having, are things we don't actually want, not when we look at what's truly important to us.

In between swigs of sweetened green tea, L told me how, in reality, success or 'what we should be' is completely different from person to person. There is no one-size-fits-all solution for what you should be doing with your life. So, to compare what you have to another person is only going to lead you to being unhappy.

With all that in mind, maybe we should just compare ourselves to who we were yesterday, rather than who anyone else is today?

And know that, as my friend L told me that day, 'You are exactly where you are meant to be.'

I Don't Want To Settle

It was just a bad day.
That doesn't mean it's a bad life.

It doesn't mean you're now forever in that darkness
locked with the hard parts you despise.
It doesn't mean
you'll wake up with the same weight on your chest
as you cry soft tears from your eyes.

It doesn't mean all of your choices are wrong.

It was just a bad day.

That's why we can turn over a new leaf
or why there's two sides to every coin.
I saw a bad day and I smiled.

It was a chance to appreciate the good ones all the more.

Dan Whitlam

Here's starting to feel like home.
Starting to feel like a setting I could settle down in
or a little place to call my own.
A new chapter, a new phase.
Blue ink for a new page.
But
that doesn't mean I've forgotten
my friends and family along the way.

It just
means I took a step down my own path
in order to find myself again.

Needed a shake-up of my last life.
Was caught in the past I
lived a week like a cycle
the days inside went too fast my

head was spinning. Falling off.
Didn't feel like I was doing enough.
But here every minute feels like it's whole and filled up.

I found myself here. In these new four walls.

I Don't Want To Settle

And though parts of my heart are back home
I know you'll understand it when I call.
That although I've left
that doesn't mean I'm forever gone.
I'm just walking down my own path, for now
to follow a new sun.

Dan Whitlam

 Look at you, doing better.
Doing better now you left a mind that was clouded by grey weather and
found yourself again.

And look how far you've come.
Past those darker days when you'd stay in bed but now you rise to a warmer sun.
I felt that too.
Like, there was nothing new.
Saying: 'This is what I am, I'm holding on to feeling blue.'

But look at you now.
Despite it all you took a different direction.
You smiled and softly walked towards that place of self-love you like to call person affection.

I found myself in a clouded mind.
And later found the sun peeping through
as it softly said:

It will only get better if you just keep doing you.

I Don't Want To Settle

☆ You're new here.
So, let me give you a few words of advice:
If you're struggling,
talking to others will always help you grow.

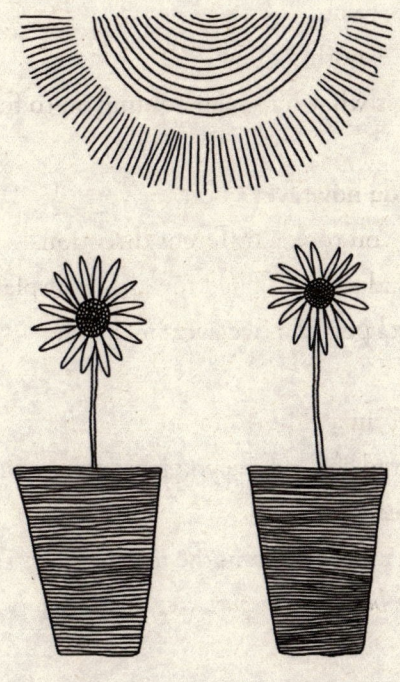

Dan Whitlam

Look at you. Healing.
Just when you thought it wasn't possible you
dropped your losses and softly called that you're done grieving.

You're done seeing yourself as someone who'll never move on.
And so you picked up the little pieces of your past self and held on
to what you hold true to you
and just look at you.

Further along than you thought, even if it's just a step or two.
A better you
who lets you do whatever's best for you.

So I guess it's true
that we're stronger than we ever imagined.

And
so on those grey days where you feel you're a little further from being healed
know that there's a person in the mirror who's slowly figured how you feel
and found the fact that
you're a being made of stardust.
And it's about time that you realised how powerful
your space really is.

I Don't Want To Settle

 She was wary of living her life in the waiting room.
Watching the clock for 'her time to come'.
A room
painted in eggshell promises that she would be happier in the future.

Happier when she got the new job. The new partner.
The home she always wanted that's slightly bigger than her neighbours'.

Happier in a future life.
Never to realise that all she needed was right here. In front of her all this time.
'A provisional life is a wasted one'.
So trade the waiting room
for a living room.
The room where you're exactly where you're supposed to be.
Filled with the dreams you had years before
and all the possibility of the next moment.

Dan Whitlam

And despite it all, you're still standing.
You took what life handed.
And found a way to go again,
through the pain and the panic
you're a fighter
who found a way to beat the fear.
Even through your darker days, and feeling lost
you can say:
'Look, world, I'm still here.'
You're still here finding the best in a bad day, a bad week.
You keep searching the world
to find roses in a garden full of weeds.
You chased pavements to find the cracks and what warmth
lies underneath.

You find the best of it all. Because you keep on going.
Despite it all. Through feeling lost you know in your heart
for certain
that you're exactly where you're meant to be. So with
courage say it clear:

'That despite it all I'm still standing.

Look, Mum, I'm still here.'

I Don't Want To Settle

You like who you're becoming.
This newer side of yourself who now gets up to let the sun
in.

Who gets up with a smile now cos you know that you found
something
that's true.
You found you like who you're becoming cos
you know that it's the real you.
The one who's a little more confident. A little more curious
and able.
Found on them spring nights, or the warmer days of April.

Just
found in your fountain pen
as you wrote soft songs about when
you'd speak dreams and then reach them
at the heights where mountains end.

You like who you're becoming
and I can see it in your eyes
a little blue on the back burner that's come alight overnight.
So when you take a drag of your cigarette and blow smoke
for a new day
know that you like who you're becoming
and I can see it too in every little way.

Dan Whitlam

You don't walk slow
through the cold bite of a night because they had to go.

You walk slow
because you're forever warmed
by that person's afterglow.

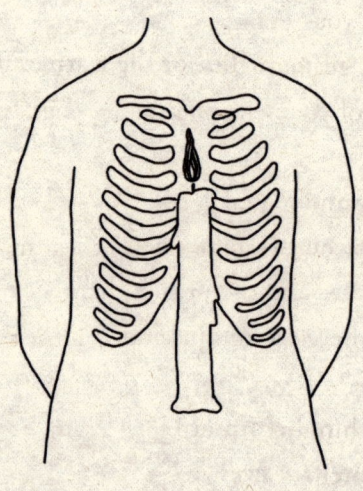

I Don't Want To Settle

 It's hard moving on
having to forget someone
in order to find yourself.

The partner you wrote in for so long, now placed back on the shelf.
To collect dust with the others.
Your collection of lovers.
Each book a little shorter than the last.
You settled for black and white. The simple stuff.
The basic bio of your being.
Said you'll never get hurt by love again.
So you give less of yourself to lessen feelings.

You stopped dreaming about it.
Stuck to the same cycle saying they'll never match up to the first.
They've ruined me for anyone else so I'll just think of them until it hurts.
It's better than thinking I could love again
now what's it worth?

It's hard moving on.
But, it's only a matter of time
before someone picks up a pen to write delicate letters
down the pages of your spine.

Dan Whitlam

 Don't mistake red flags for flowers.

To heal at the feet of those who hurt you is a step into the shade.

Heal in the light
then watch as you bloom in it too.

Find someone who picks you roses
for just being you.

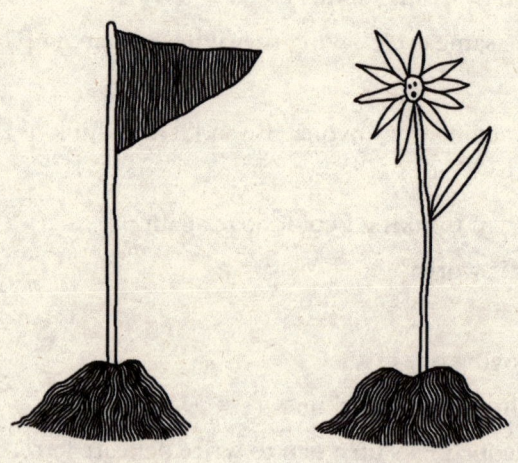

I Don't Want To Settle

 'Maybe she left so you could appreciate
what's it's like to love yourself?'

'But she's the only reason that made me want to love myself.
And now she's gone
I feel more broken than when she first found me.'

'Maybe she was teaching you that you can't rely
on other people.
If only you have your pieces
only you can put yourself back together.'

Dan Whitlam

I took a walk with myself the other day.
It wasn't extremely long but there was a warmth in the air
that seemed to say it might be nice to stretch your legs for a
little while.

We headed out on the familiar loop,
the same one I'd been doing for so many years.
Filled with potholes and flowers.
Overfilled bins and polished stone.
Past the burnt-down house that
rumour has it is not receiving its insurance payout.
The red dog collar on the park gate
begging the question of where Lucky has ran off to.

I asked myself if I was happy.
A question I rarely asked myself in fear
it might envelop me and lead to a spiral of existential crisis
swaddled in my duvet eating a gallon of pralines and cream
before
calling it a night.

I am happy, I told myself.
Well, not always. You can't always be happy.
And perhaps that's just life.
I think that's what we've learnt.
We've learnt that instead of thinking a bad day means your

I Don't Want To Settle

life is ruined
you now acknowledge it's just a day and that tomorrow or
next week will be better.
But on the whole I am happy.
A few days of pralines and cream, sure
but, you're a positive person.

I asked myself: 'What makes us smile?'

That question alone brought me to one, but I did stop for a
minute to think.
The obvious answers came pouring into my head:
Family. Friends. Being around loved ones.
Laughter. Animals. Dogs in particular.
Schnauzers with their little beards like a wise old man.
Rain. Rain in the heat of summer causing a rainbow
that everyone can't resist taking a photograph of and then
questioning what might be on the other side.
Being cold and then crawling under a warm duvet. A bed
picnic.
I realised it's ultimately the simplest of things.
It's the ordinary that makes us smile
not the big materialistic prizes.
Moments that come for free but oh how we'd pay to
experience them again and again.

Dan Whitlam

I asked myself: 'What we can improve upon?'

Silently, I want to say we're improving every day.
Just by being here and showing up we are doing enough.
It may not be hugely apparent, but just by taking a walk
and questioning ourselves
we are further along
than we were five years ago.
So maybe it's not about improvement
maybe it's just about the continuation.
We return to the same loop.
The one we've continued to walk time and time again
past the burnt-down house and the dog collar.

And it's not about doing it quicker or thinking better along the way
but maybe it's about just showing up.
Improving our life by continuing to be there for ourselves
when all we want to do is
curl up into a ball and eat pralines and cream.

I Don't Want To Settle

Whenever I've found myself a little lost
a little tired and low
a little too full of why, when and must I?
I've taken myself for a walk.
I've asked myself these three simple questions and sat with
the answers.

I hope when you're a little lost you might go for a walk too.
Sit with the answers and hopefully and in the end you'll
find that
in fact, you're
Lucky.

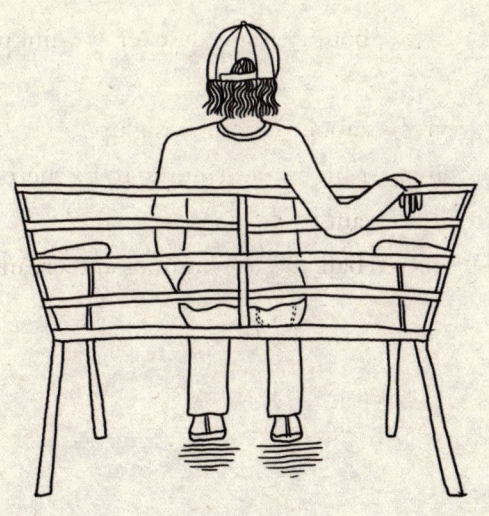

Acknowledgements

There are so many people that have contributed in some way to the writing and making of this book. While naming them all would be near impossible, there are a few I would like to mention.

My family: David, Lily, Sarah. Thank you for putting up with me and being eternally there. Lucy and the wider team from Bonnier, thank you for your trust and support. My agents, Ciara and Rosie. The Yellow Jackets. My day ones. Laurence Mitchell. Poppy Billderbeck, for your unwavering support and connection. Sean Brosnan for keeping me level-headed throughout this whirlwind of a career so far. The whole Material Music family. A massive thank you to Natti Shiner for beautifully illustrating this book. To James Coates for all your support and advice and Kate, Abi and Issy for taking a leap of faith all those years ago. Thank you to my nearest and dearest. You know who you are and I hope I tell you enough. Hannah, I'm thinking of you and I always will.

And biggest thank you to you for reading this. If you're feeling lost, you are not alone. We're all in this together.

Thank you to everyone who has supported me on this journey. Much more to come.

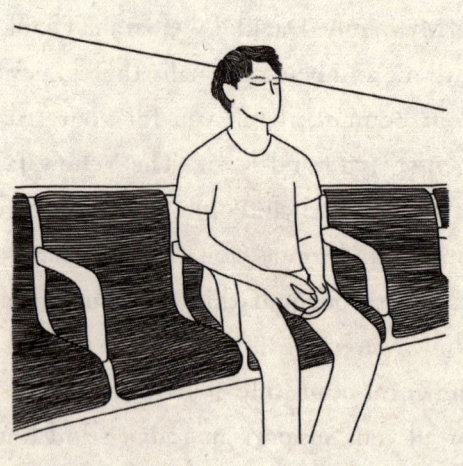